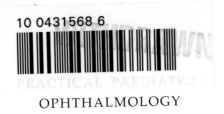
PRACTICAL PAEDIATRIC

OPHTHALMOLOGY

DATE DUE FOR RETURN

This book may be recalled before the above date.

Practical Paediatric Ophthalmology

David Taylor FRCS
& Creig Hoyt MD

b

Blackwell
Science

© 1997 by
Blackwell Science Ltd
Editorial Offices:
Osney Mead, Oxford OX2 0EL
25 John Street, London WC1N 2BL
23 Ainslie Place, Edinburgh EH3 6AJ
238 Main Street, Cambridge
 Massachusetts 02142, USA
54 University Street, Carlton
 Victoria 3053, Australia

Other Editorial Offices:
Arnette Blackwell SA
 224, Boulevard Saint Germain
 75007 Paris, France

Blackwell Wissenschafts-Verlag GmbH
 Kurfürstendamm 57
 10707 Berlin, Germany

 Zehetnergasse 6
 A-1140 Wien
 Austria

First published 1997

Set by Excel Typesetters, Hong Kong
Printed and bound in Italy
by G. Canale, SpA, Turin.

The Blackwell Science logo is a
trade mark of Blackwell Science Ltd,
registered at the United Kingdom
Trade Marks Registry

DISTRIBUTORS

Marston Book Services Ltd
PO Box 269
Abingdon
Oxon OX14 4YN
(*Orders:* Tel: 01235 465500
       Fax: 01235 465555)

USA
Blackwell Science, Inc.
238 Main Street
Cambridge, MA 02142
(*Orders:* Tel: 800 215-1000
        617 876-7000
       Fax: 617 492-5263)

Canada
Copp Clark Professional
200 Adelaide Street West, 3rd Floor
Toronto, Ontario M5H 1W7
(*Orders:* Tel: 416-597-1616
        1-800-815-9417
       Fax: 416-597-1617)

Australia
Blackwell Science Pty Ltd
54 University Street
Carlton, Victoria 3053
(*Orders:* Tel: 03 9347 0300
       Fax: 03 9349 3016)

A catalogue record for this title
is available from the British Library

ISBN 0-86542-720-8

Library of Congress
Cataloging-in-publication Data

Taylor, David, 1942–
 Practical paediatric ophthalmology/
 David Taylor, Creig Hoyt.
   p.   cm.
 Includes bibliographical references
and index.
 ISBN 0-86542-720-8
 1 Pediatric ophthalmology.
I Hoyt, Creig Simmons, 1942–
II Title.
 [DNLM: 1 Eye Diseases—in infancy &
childhood. WW 600
T239p 1997]
RE48.2.C5T39   1997
618.92'0977—dc20
DNLM/DLC
for Library of Congress
                          96-18413
                          CIP

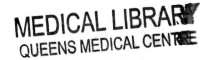

Contents

Preface

We hope that this book will help ophthalmologists and others to help their child patients and their parents. It is a distillation of our experience and, although written in a compact style, we hope that it will be an easy read and a ready source of information. We believe that paediatric ophthalmology and strabismus are inseparable disciplines and we hope that the nearly conjoined twin of this book, *Practical Strabismus Management* by Vivian and Morris (Blackwell Science, 1997) will be used to help those patients with strabismus. We have included only essential discussion and no references in order to keep the book compact. A much more detailed and referenced analysis of every area covered in this book is to be found in *Paediatric Ophthalmology* (2nd edn, Blackwell Science, 1997).

We wrote this book in a week-long burst of intense activity in London and Paris, helped by Angela Tank, Jo Wilby, Anna Taylor and Mathew Taylor. After being on the road for 7 years, Jack Kerouac wrote *On the Road* in 3 weeks; whilst not claiming any similarity to that literary thoroughbred, we can claim a parallel intensity of enjoyment in the preparation and writing. We sincerely hope that those who purchase this book will also find it not only useful but enjoyable.

David Taylor
Creig Hoyt

1: Introduction

Since one-third of ophthalmology patients in the West are children and since there are about 1.5 million severely visually impaired or blind children throughout the world and many of these have genetic disease, it is natural that the study of children's eyes and the treatment of abnormalities arising in the eyes and visual system has become a separate speciality in its own right. There is an artificial distinction in many countries between paediatric ophthalmology and strabismus management. This is historical but plainly ridiculous because, although it is inevitable that some specialists will develop a greater interest in certain aspects, strabismus, being the most common form of eye problem in childhood and occurring in very many children with eye and systemic disease, falls within the remit of any paediatric ophthalmologist. It would similarly be fatuous to suggest that an ophthalmologist should just develop an interest in paediatric ophthalmology whilst ignoring strabismus, or in strabismus whilst ignoring the non-ocular features of these conditions.

Blindness has a devastating effect on a child because it is lifelong and it affects all areas of development, therefore the significance of 1.5 million blind children in the world is much greater than it appears at first sight.

The paediatric ophthalmologist not only has to have a knowledge of a special set of diseases but he/she needs to have a different way of approaching clinical examination, history taking and management to any other ophthalmologist. A formal approach is not usually successful. The paediatric ophthalmologist needs to make the child feel 'at home' even after such unpleasant procedures as putting in eyedrops. He/she needs to have a great deal of compassion and understanding of the family background and the sort of things that make life difficult for children, their parents and indeed the whole family.

Epidemiology

There were 1.5 million severely visually impaired and blind children in the world in 1992. These children are blind for life, so in blind-years terms this is a very significant figure. Fifty per cent of blind children die in childhood. In Canada the incidence of congenital blindness is three per 10 000 live births.

Causes
1 Developed world.
   (a) Genetic disease:
     (i) retina;
     (ii) cataract;
     (iii) glaucoma.
   (b) Intrauterine infections.
   (c) Acquired disease:
     (i) retinopathy of prematurity;
     (ii) cortical visual impairment;
     (iii) trauma;
     (iv) infections (rare);
     (v) cataract.
2 Developing world.
   (a) Malnutrition—avitaminosis A.
   (b) Genetic disease:
     (i) retina;
     (ii) lens;
     (iii) measles infection;
     (iv) traditional medications.
3 Intermediate countries. Retinopathy of prematurity increasingly significant.

Screening

Screening may be defined as the economical detection of presymptomatic disease. It is important to realise that screening cannot be 100% effective. It is inevitable that there will be a number of false positives and false negatives. Screening programmes need to fulfil these criteria.

1 The condition must be a significant health problem to the individual or the community.

2 The natural history of the condition must be known.

3 A latent or preclinical phase must exist.

4 An effective treatment must be available.

5 The screening test should be simple, inexpensive, non-invasive and acceptable to the population.

6 The screening test must be valid, with reasonable levels of specificity and sensitivity.

7 Full diagnostic and therapeutic services must be available.

8 Early intervention must favourably influence the outcome.

9 The screening programme should be cost-effective.

10 The screening programme should be continuous.

Screening for amblyopia and squint

Screening for amblyopia and squint is still contentious because: (i) being a unilateral condition the child's life or general health is not seriously threatened; (ii) the treatment does not always work (compliance with occlusion is the main cause for this); and (iii) screening for it can be an expensive procedure.

Methods of screening

1 *Screening at birth* effectively only detects gross abnormalities of the external eye, and screening by the use of ophthalmoscope detects media opacities only. Refractive errors and fundus abnormalities are not usually detected because screening is carried out by non-ophthalmologists.

2 *Vision tests at 3.5 years of age.* This is useful but detects the condition when it is relatively resistant to treatment, at an age when it is difficult to start patching because compliance is low. Tests by paramedical staff can be effective if they are well trained.

3 *Screening for amblyogenic factors.* Refractive error and squint can be screened by paramedical staff using photorefraction and simple tests.

4 *School screening.* Vision is tested in many schools in the developed world. The tester is usually a school nurse or teacher and patients falling below defined levels of acuity, for example 6/9 or 20/30, are either retested or referred if the acuity is 6/12, 20/40 or worse. Near and distance tests should be carried out. Amblyopia detected at this age may be untreatable.

5 *Screening should be undertaken for high-risk groups* such as those children with a family history of cataract, aniridia, retinoblastoma, etc.

6 *Screening for retinopathy of prematurity.* Since it has been shown that retinopathy of prematurity can be favourably influenced by cryotherapy or laser treatment, screening has now become mandatory in most countries (see Chapter 17).

7 *Screening for infectious diseases.* This is much more controversial. For instance, screening for toxoplasmosis is resisted in many countries where the criteria for screening are not fulfilled, i.e. for toxoplasmosis the treatment is not 100% risk-free. The natural history is not well known, i.e. the amount of damage to an affected fetus is very variable and unpredictable. Therefore, early intervention does not necessarily favourably influence the outcome. In many countries where the incidence of toxoplasmosis is very high, screening may be more effective.

The significance of visual defects

Childhood visual defects have an impact way beyond their effects on the visual system alone.

1 There may be associated systemic disease.

2 Other spheres of general development are delayed, for example:
  (a) speech delay;
  (b) difficulty in relating to parents, other children and other family members;
  (c) autism;
  (d) stereotyped behaviour, i.e. repetitive, purposeless movements, eye poking, rocking, etc.;
  (e) impaired intellectual potential;
  (f) learning difficulties;
  (g) delayed motor development, hypotonia and weakness;
  (h) obesity.

Mental retardation is present in a high proportion of blind children, and a significant proportion of mentally handicapped children have an associated visual defect.

Early intervention

It has been shown that early positive management of the blind child and his/her family, including advice to the parents on early stimulation, the provision of appropriate stimulating toys, provision of appropriate furniture, i.e. a chair which the child can sit in and see his/her surroundings from (using any residual vision), and giving parents detailed guidance of the handling of the child, is beneficial.

Box 1.1 The newly diagnosed blind infant

1 Get the diagnosis right for the following reasons:
   (a) genetics;
   (b) management.
2 Delay full discussion until diagnosis is certain.
3 Always give interim information and plan of action.
4 Repeat interviews and discussions are mandatory. Remember that most intelligent people can only take in a very few pieces of new information at a time.
5 Give simple explanations with diagrams, pictures and models. Be honest about how much and how little you know.
6 If no treatment possible, explain why.
7 Explain the prognosis in functional terms.
   (a) How the child will navigate in the future?
   (b) Will normal education be possible?
   (c) Will driving be possible?
8 Get a second opinion if necessary.
9 Define blindness and visually handicapped for the parents.
10 Stimulate any residual vision, arrange early intervention.
11 Never be overpessimistic about the visual prognosis.
12 Think about other handicaps:
   (a) mental retardation;
   (b) deafness;
   (c) others.
13 Allow the parents to take notes or tape the discussion.

Box 1.2 The family of the visually handicapped baby

1 Parents:
   (a) slowly realise the enormity of the problem;
   (b) early advice necessary;
   (c) simple support measures;
   (d) parents groups;
   (e) disease groups, i.e. neurofibromatosis, tuberous sclerosis, etc., societies;
   (f) babysitting;
   (g) home help;
   (h) help with home appliances, etc.
2 Siblings:
   (a) avoid jealousy due to the family resources being concentrated on the handicapped child;
   (b) the parents should remember they are just as important as the handicapped baby/child;
   (c) family resources need to be evenly distributed.
3 Grandparents:
   (a) often profoundly disturbed by visual handicap in a grandchild, and thus need to be involved;
   (b) can be very useful for babysitting and other help to relieve pressure on parents.

2: Development of the Eye and Vision

The visual systems of the newborn infant are not adult-like. Both the ocular and neural structures essential for vision will undergo anatomical and physiological changes as part of the maturation process. Maturation of all the visual systems occurs relatively rapidly in the normal child, albeit at somewhat different rates.

Visual acuity in the preverbal child may be assessed using several different techniques.

1 *Behavioural assessment*: the standard clinical technique utilizes evaluation of fixation and following behaviour under both monocular and binocular conditions. Normal visual development is considered to proceed as follows:

(a) steady fixation—6 weeks;
(b) fixation and following—2 months;
(c) visual directed reaching—4 months;
(d) small hand/eye co-ordinated tasks—1 year.

2 Optokinetic nystagmus techniques may also be utilized in the assessment of visual acuity but have essentially been replaced by forced preferential looking (FPL) or visual evoked potential (VEP) techniques:

(a) acuity at birth up to 6/60 (20/200).
(b) development of 6/6 (20/20) by 3–4 years.

3 *FPL*. This technique is predicated on the observation that the developing child would prefer to look at a patterned stimulus rather than a homogeneous luminance-controlled comparable one. Assessment with this technique documents normal development as follows:

(a) acuity at birth—6/36 to 6/60;
(b) development of 6/6 by 3 years of age or more.

4 *VEP*. This technique, utilizing a pattern stimulus for measurement of cortical responses, provides the most rapid maturation data of any of the acuity assessment techniques:

(a) acuity at birth—6/24 to 6/36.
(b) development of 6/6 acuity by 6–8 months.

5 *Recognition acuity*. Under most circumstances clinicians consider standard techniques of recognition acuity (Snellen line or single letter) to be the gold standard for visual acuity assessment.

(a) Acuity at 4 years old—6/6 to 6/12.
(b) By 7 years of age 70% of normals will achieve 6/6.

Binocularity

Normal binocularity does not exist at birth. Different techniques have been utilized to assess its normal maturation. All of these tests suggest that binocularity is normally established within the first few months of life.

- Stereoacuity achieved: 2–6 months.
- Ocular motor fusion developed: 3–6 months.

At birth some degree of immaturity is present in all visual structures and important neural pathways. Maturation of these systems normally occurs relatively rapidly.

Retina

Both anatomical and functional changes occur in the first few months of life in a normal infant. This may be seen in the normal changes that occur in electroretinographic (ERG) recordings. Thus, the amplitude of photopic responses of the ERG increase rapidly in the first few months of life. Morphologically, differentiation of rods and cones can be identified during the second trimester of pregnancy. In contrast, normal foveal development does not occur until post-natally and may continue to show maturational changes for up to 5 years. In general the peripheral retina appears more mature at birth than the central retina. Migration of rods from the central portion of the retina to the periphery as well as cones from the midperipheral retina to the central is a normal post-natal event that may go on for more than 1 year. Maturation of the normal vasculature of the retina is, of course, important in understanding the pathogenesis of retinopathy of prematurity and some other disorders of retinal vasculature. Vascularization of the temporal retina is ordinarily not complete until 44 weeks gestational age.

Optic nerve and anterior visual pathways

Neuronal development in what will be the normal optic nerve can be identified in the first trimester of gestational development. At birth an excessive number of neurones in the anterior visual pathway may be identified. As a result, cellular death of a large percentage of these neurones is a normal development phenomena (apoptosis). This production of excessive neurones may be an attempt of the developing system to provide a strategy for recovery from injuries to the developing pathways. Although myelination of the anterior visual pathways can be identified early in development, complete myelination does not occur until 2 years following birth. This may be assessed by standard magnetic resonance imaging (MRI) studies.

Refractive state and growth of the eye

Changes in the axial length of the eye, corneal curvature and thickness of the crystalline lens are normal developmental processes in infancy. Thus, the axial length of the eye at birth is usually 16–17 mm and does not approach the normal adult measurement until 1–2 years of age. The corneal curvature of the newborn infant is much steeper than in adults and this makes contact lens fitting for the aphakic infant difficult. Increased thickness of the crystalline lens occurs as a normal process with age. It should not be surprising that transient refractive errors may occur as the result of these normal developmental changes of the structures essential in the refractive process. Thus, for example, a significant percentage of infants will show astigmatism in the first year of life which will subsequently not be apparent as the child matures.

By far the most dramatic developmental changes occur in the visual cortex and associated cortex areas essential for vision. Cortical neuronal dendritic growth and synaptic formation begin as a normal process at approximately 25 weeks gestational age. These continue until at least 2 years of age post-natally. Maturation of the VEP correlates best with the degree of dendritic formation of the visual cortex. Segregation of the ocular dominance columns, so essential in understanding the anatomical changes that occur in amblyopia, usually occurs at or near birth.

Delayed visual maturation

This term applies to a group of children who present with visual development poorer than would be expected for their chronological age. The simplistic notion has been that these children represent a delay in the normal maturation of one or more of the visual systems. Almost certainly this is an oversimplified view of what is occurring in this group of children. The essential features of this condition are considered to be the following:
1 poor visual fixation and following for age;
2 no nystagmus;
3 normal ophthalmological examination;
4 no evidence of cortical visual impairment.
Whilst it is generally true that this subgroup of children subsequently develop normal visual function, many are found to have a mild to moderate neurological or developmental problem on subsequent evaluations. A system of categories for children with delayed visual maturation has been proposed as follows.
• *Group 1*: isolated anomaly.
• *Group 2*: those in whom obvious and persistent neurological and developmental anomalies are noted.
• *Group 3*: those who have ocular abnormalities presumably related to the development of delayed visual maturation, i.e. cataract or albinism.

Investigation of these patients may be carried out utilizing standard visual assessment and neural imaging techniques. Thus, in most cases these tests will demonstrate the following:
• FPL—usually very poor;

- VEP (pattern)—often near normal;
- computerized tomography (CT) or MRI scanning —no major defects.

It is still not apparent what the anatomical and physiological correlates are for delayed visual maturation. Improvement nonetheless occurs in most cases.

Amblyopia

Definition

Whilst no all encompassing definition for amblyopia is possible, the term generally refers to the reduction in visual acuity that occurs as the result of interruption of normal visual development during a so-called 'sensitive' period. If the problem is identified during the 'sensitive' period it is potentially reversible. However, if not identified until the sensitive period is complete, the visual loss is permanent. For example, monocular congenital cataracts and their associated amblyopia are generally considered not to be treatable after the first several months of life.

Amblyopia is usually considered to be a unilateral visual loss but under certain circumstances it may occur bilaterally. At least five distinct forms of amblyopia may be identified based on the aetiology of the visual deprivation and whether it is unilateral or bilateral.

1 Unilateral:
  (a) form deprivation;
  (b) strabismus;
  (c) anisometropia.
2 Bilateral:
  (a) ametropic (including meridonal);
  (b) form deprivation.

Each of these forms of amblyopia is considered to have a different duration of the sensitive period. The treatability of amblyopia is therefore directly dependent upon the aetiology. Thus, strabismus and anisometropic amblyopia are treatable for several years, whereas occlusion amblyopia is treatable only for a few months.

Diagnosis

Ideally, amblyopia would be detected in all patients as the result of visual acuity measurements. Since this is not possible in many affected young children, the presence of amblyopia is usually inferred as the result of the identification of the underlying aetiological condition. For example, the detection of a monocular cataract in infancy would almost invariably imply that form deprivation amblyopia will occur. Screening of children for amblyopia therefore is geared at identifying potential amblyopic conditions.

- Early infancy: identification of a good red light reflex in each eye to rule out form deprivation amblyopia, i.e. cataract, corneal defect.
- One to 2 years of age: assessment of ocular alignment by light reflexes, cover test or photorefraction to rule out the presence of strabismus or a predisposing refractive error.
- Three to 6 years of age: recognition visual acuity screening to identify the presence of anisometropic amblyopia as well as strabismus amblyopia.

Management

Successful treatment of amblyopia requires that the abnormal visual condition be reversed and, under most circumstances, that occlusion of the fixing (non-affected) eye be undertaken. The following goals for each form of amblyopia are therefore:

1 form deprivation amblyopia—clear the visual axis by surgery;
2 strabismic amblyopia—realign the ocular axis;
3 anisometropic amblyopia—correct the refractive error.

Occlusion therapy is usually monitored by assessment of visual acuity in both the fixing and affected eye. Excessive occlusion of the fixing eye may cause occlusion amblyopia. An alternative to patching the fixing eye is penalization therapy: this utilizes cycloplegia of the fixing eye rather than occlusion. In order to be effective the fixing eye should be hyperopic and the amblyopia mild to moderate. In some circumstances it is the preferred treatment for amblyopia; for example, in the case of strabismus amblyopia in association with nystagmus. Even when amblyopia is associated with a structural lesion of the affected eye, occlusion therapy should be undertaken for a trial period.

Box 2.1 Practical patching tips

The more severe the visual loss in amblyopia, the more difficult patching therapy will initially be. Failure to complete the appropriate occlusion therapy is still a primary reason for failure in amblyopia treatment and is estimated to occur in 30–40% of cases. Although no sure-fire technique exists to assure that all children will complete an effective patching programme, the following points may be helpful in treating the child who resists occlusion therapy.

1 Be certain the parents fully understand the reason for, and the importance of, occlusion therapy. Without their wholehearted participation it is doomed to fail.

2 If the child is old enough, explain to the child why the therapy is necessary.

3 Clean the skin before using the sticky patch. Alternatively, the use of colloidal agents to protect the skin from the adhesive may be used.

4 Put the patch on whilst the child is asleep.

5 Put additional tape on top of the patch.

6 Use soft cotton mittens with a drawstring at the wrist to prevent the child from pulling the patch off.

7 Use soft elbow restraints. These may be made of cardboard or other non-abrasive materials.

8 Reward the child when successful patching is noted.

9 Re-emphasize the need for patching routinely in follow-up examinations.

3: Refractive Errors

The refractive power of the eye results from four factors and their interaction:
1 corneal steepness (power);
2 depth of anterior chamber;
3 lens power (thickness and curvature);
4 axial length of the eye.

Abnormalities of one or more of these structures may result in a significant refractive error. For example, excessive axial eye growth will usually lead to myopia.

Whilst mild degrees of hypermetropia are normal in the infant and young child, high degrees of hypermetropia, myopia or astigmatism may result in not only blurred vision, but also strabismus and amblyopia. Transient refractive errors, especially astigmatism, are common in the first year of life (Fig. 3.1).

Several techniques are available for detecting refractive errors in young children.

Visual screening

Standard screening techniques whilst utilizing recognition visual acuity measurements are aimed primarily at detecting the presence of amblyopia or high refractive errors. Regrettably, these techniques are not usually effective in children under the age of 3–4 years.

Autorefraction

In general, autorefractors are not reliable in children unless performed after cycloplegia.

Photorefraction

Photorefraction is a photographic technique that estimates the refractive error based on the reflected image of a light shined at the eye. Two different forms of photorefraction are available.
1 *On-axis photorefraction*. This technique requires several photographs to assess the refractive error and has generally been replaced by off-axis photorefraction.
2 *Off-axis photorefraction* requires only one or two photographs to assess refractive error. It is thus usually more cost-effective especially in screening programmes.

The major limitation of all photorefractive techniques is the failure to detect small refractive errors, especially hypermetropia, unless cycloplegia is utilized.

Refraction

Subjective and objective refractive techniques remain the gold standard for detecting significant refractive errors in children.

Refractive techniques

Several different techniques are available to estimate the refractive error under either cycloplegic or non-cycloplegic conditions.

Non-cycloplegic examinations: retinoscopy

1 *Subjective refraction* (fogging). By placing plus lenses in front of the eye one can prevent accommodation during subjective refraction. Thus, one always starts with more plus lenses in front of the eye than is anticipated to be the appropriate refractive prescription.
2 *Distance fixation*. One may control the fixation of the patient and be certain that they are fixating in the distance in an effort to relax accommodation. This is rarely an effective technique in children.
3 *Dynamic retinoscopy* can be performed. This is done in the dark and is primarily a research tool.

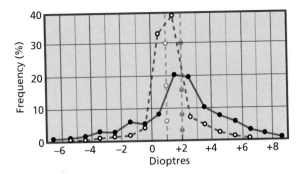

Fig. 3.1 Distribution of refraction in neonates (closed circles) and 10 year olds (open circles). (From Cook & Glasscock (1951) *Am J Ophthalmol*; **34**: 1407–13 and Fledelius (1976) *Acta Ophthalmol*; **54**: 1–243.)

Cycloplegic examination

In most circumstances cycloplegia is necessary in order to obtain a reliable refraction in children. This type of examination is done following instillation of one of several cycloplegic agents.

1 Atropine 0.5% or 1% one to three times a day for 3 days prior to examination.

2 Cyclopentolate 1% twice within 10 minutes on the day of examination. Refraction needs to be performed approximately 30–40 minutes following instillation.

3 Tropicamide 1% twice in 10 minutes on the day of examination. Refraction may be performed after approximately 30 minutes. This is the least reliable cycloplegic examination as it rarely produces complete cycloplegia, although good pupillary dilatation is usually achieved.

4 In infants cyclopentolate 0.5% or tropicamide 0.5% are used.

Subjective techniques as well as retinoscopic examinations are most accurate when done following cycloplegia.

Errors in refraction

Subjective techniques

The primary problems in subjective refractions arise as the result of failure to control accommodation. This commonly leads to the overestimation of myopic errors. Some authorities have estimated that as many as 10–15% of myopes

are routinely overcorrected in their refractive prescriptions.

Retinoscopic techniques

Although retinoscopy is seen as a more objective technique in the evaluation of refractive errors it also has limitations. The short axial length of the normal infant eye leads to overestimation of the amount of hypermetropia in the first few months of life, unless the examiner shortens his/her normal working distance. Even more important, retinoscopy performed off axis, even 10–15°, may produce an overestimation of the presence and amount of astigmatism.

Myopia

Myopia is the most frequent refractive error with a progressive course seen in most affected children. Occasionally one sees transient myopia in the early infant period.

Prevalence

Although the prevalence of myopia is at least in part dependent upon genetic and environmental factors it is also age dependent. Thus, in normal-term infants it is estimated to occur in 4–6% of cases, whereas in pre-school infants it occurs in no more than 2–3%. With increasing age, myopia is detected more frequently. Thus, in the 11–13-year-old age-group it is seen in 4% of patients, and in adults over 20 years it is estimated to be present in 25% of cases. It should be recalled that the premature child is especially prone to the development of myopia; in some reports as high as 30–50% of cases.

Myopia is an important cause of visual disability in all populations. This occurs both as the result of the refractive blur resulting from it, as well as its association with other significant ocular problems and systemic disorders.

Associated ocular findings

A number of ocular abnormalities are significantly associated with myopia. In general, the more serious of these are associated with higher degrees of myopia. Associated ocular findings include:
• chorioretinal degeneration;

- lattice degeneration;
- schisis;
- retinal detachment;
- Fuchs' spots (Fig. 3.2);
- tilted and dysplastic optic nerves (Fig. 3.3);
- glaucoma;
- vitreous degeneration and detachment;
- subretinal neovascularization;
- microcornea;
- chorioretinal and/or optic nerve colobomas (Fig. 3.4).

Systemic associations

Myopia is associated with a number of systemic disorders. When myopia is detected, especially in the young infant, these systemic associations should be recalled:

- albinism;
- Alport's syndrome;
- Alagille's syndrome;
- Bassen–Kornsweig's syndrome;
- Down's syndrome (trisomy 21);
- Ehlers–Danlos syndrome;
- Fabry's disease;
- Flynn–Aird syndrome;
- Laurence–Moon–Bardet–Biedl syndrome;
- Marfan's syndrome;
- Marshall's syndrome;
- Stickler's syndrome;
- Wagner's dystrophy;
- choroideraemia;

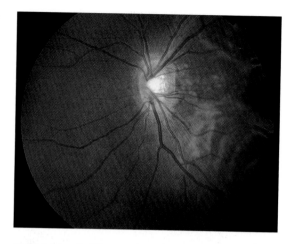

Fig. 3.3 Myopia. The optic disc is vertically oval and has peripapillary degeneration. There is a posterior staphyloma evidenced by the more visible choroidal vascular pattern and a tilting of the optic disc.

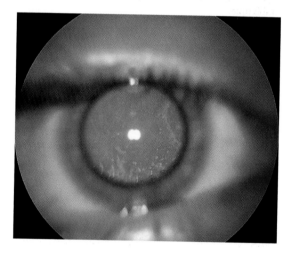

Fig. 3.4 Vitreous floaters in a highly myopic eye with posterior vitreous detachment. The fellow eye had a retinal detachment.

- ectopia lentis;
- gyrate atrophy;
- myelinated nerve fibres (Fig. 3.5);
- retinitis pigmentosa;
- retinopathy of prematurity.

Several different techniques are available for correction of refractive errors. These include:

- spectacles;

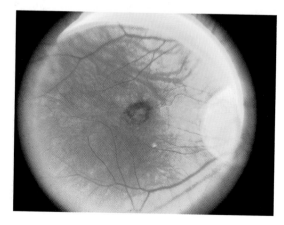

Fig. 3.2 Fuchs' spot.

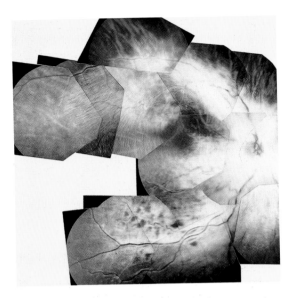

Fig. 3.5 High myopia with myelinated nerve fibres and amblyopia.

- contact lenses;
- refractive surgery — not appropriate for most children.

Several forms of therapy have been devised in an effort to prevent or halt the progression of myopia. These include:
- eye exercises—unproven;
- cycloplegic agents—remains controversial;
- bifocal lenses — conflicting results published to date;
- prisms—no evidence of effect;
- orthokeratography — hard contact lenses that sit tightly on the cornea, which produces at least a short-term effect, but long-term effects are unknown;
- scleral reinforcing injections or tissue reinforcement procedures—remain unproven.

Hypermetropia (hyperopia)

Hypermetropia is the normal state of the infant and young child's eye and comes about as the result of short axial length, small cornea, normal lens thickness and shallow anterior chamber.

Significance

If accommodation is normal, hypermetropia rarely causes symptoms in the first decade of life. As accommodation decreases in the second decade, uncorrected hypermetropia may lead to headaches and blurred vision. Its most important significance is its association with a large percentage of esodeviations.

Associated ocular findings

Hypermetropia may be associated with other ocular abnormalities especially strabismus. These include:
- strabismus (accommodative and infantile esotropia);
- nanophthalmos;
- pseudopapilloedema (Fig. 3.6);
- positive angle alpha.

Systemic associations

High degrees of hypermetropia may be associated with certain systemic abnormalities. These include:
- albinism;
- Franceschetti's syndrome (microphthalmos, macrophakia, tapetal retinal degeneration);
- Leber's congenital amaurosis;
- autosomal dominant retinitis pigmentosa.

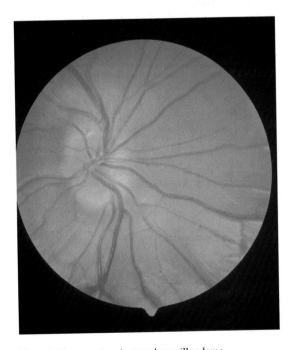

Fig. 3.6 Hypermetropic pseudopapilloedema.

Management

Young children with small degrees of hypermetropia and no strabismus do not usually require any refractive correction. Children with hypermetropia and strabismus (esotropia) usually require a full cycloplegic hypermetropic refractive correction in order to assess its effect on the strabismic deviation. In older children with symptoms of blur and headache, hypermetropic correction for the symptoms should be prescribed. Whether unrecognized hypermetropia in pre-school children contributes to school learning disabilities remains controversial. Also controversial is the theory that uncorrected hypermetropia in infancy leads to strabismus.

Astigmatism

There is a high prevalence of astigmatism in normal infants. It should be recalled, however, that off-axis retinoscopy may contribute to an overdetection of astigmatism in infancy. Astigmatism generally diminishes during the first year of life. After 8 years of age little change in refractive astigmatism is seen in most patients who do not have associated corneal pathologies (e.g. keratoconus).

Significance

Astigmatism is important in its association with amblyopia and strabismus. A number of associated ocular problems may occur with astigmatism. These include:
- corneal pathology (including keratoconus);
- optic nerve hypoplasia;
- ptosis;
- congenital motor nystagmus.

Some systemic abnormalities have also been associated with significant degrees of astigmatism. These include:
- albinism;
- fetal alcohol syndrome;
- retinitis pigmentosa.

The management of astigmatism is usually not difficult when it is regular and of low powers. The astigmatism may be treated by:
- spectacle correction;
- contact lenses/gas permeable or toric soft;
- refractive surgery techniques—usually inappropriate for children.

4: History, Examination and Further Investigations

General eye history

Although it is true that one generally does not take as detailed a history when examining a young infant or child, it is important not to forget to obtain a sufficiently detailed history. The following questions should be addressed.

1 Have the parents or paediatrician noted any specific problem with the child's eyes?
2 Was the child premature? Was the peri-natal period normal?
3 Does the child have any systemic abnormality?
4 Is the child taking any medication?
5 Does the child have any systemic illnesses or abnormalities?
6 Have any problems of general eye health been noted? For example, does the child have excessive tearing, chronic redness, unequal pupils, etc.?
7 Does the child's ocular or visual development differ in any significant way from his/her siblings?

Family history

Many disorders that are important in the young child are genetically inherited. It is important to obtain a detailed family history. The following points should be addressed.

1 Does anyone in the family have a similar ocular problem?
2 Does anyone in the family have significant eye problems even if they are apparently different from the patient's?
3 Are the mother and father related?
4 Are there any diseases that seem to run through the family even if they are not apparently associated with ocular problems?

Vision history

Most of the time devoted to obtaining a history of the child's health will be directed to assessing visual development. Questions that may be helpful to answer are the following.

1 How well does the child see?
2 Is the visual behaviour of the child different from his/her siblings?
3 Are any abnormal problems about the patient's vision noted? For example, is the child photophobic?
4 How have the general developmental milestones that are vision dependent progressed? Is there any evidence of general motor development delay?

If a visual difficulty is noted it is important to ascertain if there is any variability in this difficulty. Variability may occur either:

1 in time, i.e. the child seems to have good and bad days, a common finding in the cortically visually impaired child; or
2 depending on changes in the visual environment — for example, the patient with a cone dystrophy will be photophobic and prefer to avoid a brightly lit room.

General eye examination

Visual behaviour and acuity assessment
Observation
In almost all cases this is the most important part of the examination. One can usually quickly note whether or not the child fixes and follows during the history-taking process. Visual fixation should be steady and following movements smooth and in the appropriate direction of the target of interest. It should be noted that the ability to follow a visual target (as usually tested clinically) is usually dependent on normal saccadic movements (not pursuit),

and in many neurologically handicapped children this ability is impaired. Therefore, the failure to fix and follow should not always be equated with visual loss. Similarly, children with significant visual impairment of one or both eyes may generate reasonably normal fixation and following movements.

Fixation testing

Assessment of fixation may be refined by utilizing the CSM system pioneered by R.F. Zipf (1976). This is an assessment of whether each eye can fixate centrally, steadily and maintain fixation. Note that assessment of central and steady fixation is done under monocular viewing conditions. For example, one occludes the left eye and evaluates if the right eye fixates on a target centrally and then steadily (no nystagmoid movements being noted) for a few seconds. One then allows the patient to view the target under binocular circumstances. If the tested eye maintains its fixation on the target, one assumes that visual acuity in this eye is normal. On the other hand, if the examined eye under binocular viewing conditions immediately deviates and the patient takes up fixation with the previously occluded eye, the visual acuity in the tested eye is assumed to be abnormal. One should note that whilst this is a good test for detection of diminished visual acuity, it is a poor quantitative test. Central study unmaintained fixation may be seen in an eye with visual acuity from 6/9 to 6/36. Moreover, this test cannot be performed in the patient without strabismus since the assessment of maintained fixation will be meaningless if the eyes are well aligned.

Prism test

In order to assess the patient with no strabismus the 10-Dioptre (10-D) vertical prism test is utilized. A 10-D prism is introduced either base down or base up in front of one eye. This will induce a vertical strabismus, usually, of 10 D. The normal response is for the eye without the prism in front of it to take up fixation. If the eye with the prism in front of it fixates this is an abnormal response and suggests that the eye without the prism has reduced visual acuity.

Objective quantification

Three techniques have been utilised to objectively quantitate visual function in the preliterate child. These are optokinetic nystagmus, forced choice preferential looking and visually evoked potentials.

Optokinetic nystagmus

Although optokinetic nystagmus techniques were historically the first ones to be developed, they are rarely utilized today.

Forced choice preferential looking

Forced choice preferential looking techniques are based upon the notion that the child's visual system would prefer to see a visual environment with pattern to it rather than a homogeneous patternless one. Thus, if one shows a child a set of vertically orientated stripes in the right visual field and a homogeneous luminance-controlled target in the left visual field, if the child's visual system can resolve the vertical lines of the test target, the child will preferentially look to his/her right. This test may be done under monocular or binocular viewing conditions. It is currently available in a portable series of cards known as the Teller or Keeler Cards (Fig. 4.1).

One should note that assessment of visual function by this test requires an ocular motor as well as head and neck movement response. Failure of the child to respond to this test may be due to a problem

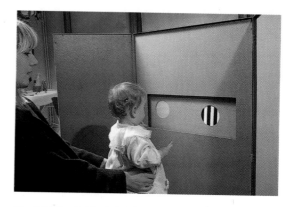

Fig. 4.1 The child is being tested with a forced choice preferential technique. One would expect the child to look toward the pattern stimulus.

of the ocular motor system rather than the primary sensory system. Moreover, this test has a tendency to overestimate the visual acuity in certain pathological conditions (most importantly, in all forms of amblyopia).

Visual evoked potentials

Visual evoked potentials have the advantage that no ocular motor response is necessary in order to obtain an estimate of visual function. Visual attention, however, is imperative if artifacts are not to be introduced into this testing. The visual stimulus used for this form of visual evoked potential must be patterned rather than a simple flash. Since it, too, is an assessment of grating visual acuity it may overestimate the visual function in the amblyopic eye. It should also be noted that the exact source of the waveforms measured in visual evoked potentials is not known.

Optotype testing

A variety of Snellen visual acuity and other optotypes are available for assessment of visual function even in the young child. The standard Snellen visual acuity chart is the gold standard, but other tests available include Landolt C rings, numbers, child-recognition test (picture optotypes) and the so-called E Game. An attempt should be made to obtain visual acuity assessment at both near and distance fixation. It should be recalled that the

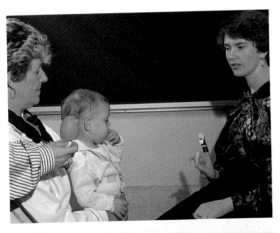
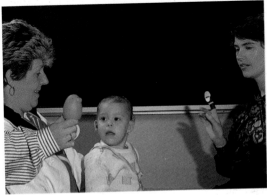

Fig. 4.3 This young child's peripheral field is being tested with a colourful toy. One expects the child to move the head and eyes to the target if no field defect exists.

amblyopic eye performs better when tested with isolated targets. Thus, whenever possible a full line of letter acuity should be used in the assessment of amblyopia.

Visual fields

Although it is not possible to perform ordinary computerised perimetric visual field examinations in young children, these may be successfully performed in most school age children (Fig. 4.2). Confrontation techniques may be used at all ages. Utilizing interesting colourful targets, one may ascertain whether or not a child appears to make saccadic movements in the appropriate direction of the target in the peripheral visual field (Fig. 4.3). One should recall that the patient with a congenital

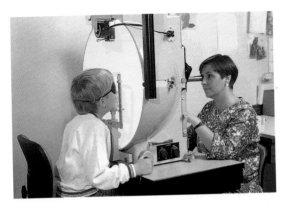

Fig. 4.2 This young boy is having a Goldmann field test performed. The Humphrey Field Analyser or other computerised techniques are more commonly used today.

hemifield defect may make saccadic movements into the blind field but that these are usually hypometric. Electrophysiological techniques may be helpful in certain special circumstances. It should not be forgotten that in congenital hemianopia, trans-synaptic degeneration of the neurovisual pathways may be identified by inspection of the optic nerve.

Colour vision

Colour vision testing may be useful in assessing optic nerve or retinal dysfunction. It may be performed with a number of standardized colour plates (e.g. Ishihara, City University, Llantony or HRR) or with matching tests such as the Farnsworth D15. The inability to name colours, frequently seen in young children, should not be misinterpreted to imply that the child is colour blind (Fig. 4.4).

Pupils

Inspection of the pupil size, configuration and reactivity to light and/or darkness is an important part of the ocular examination in children.

Afferent system

The afferent loop of the pupillary light response is the retinal and neural pathways connected to the pretectal brainstem region.

Efferent system

The efferent pathways include the third cranial nerve as well as the sympathetic system.

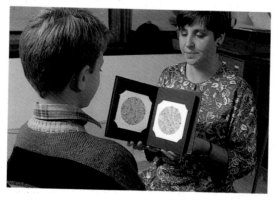

Fig. 4.4 This child is identifying the Ishihara test plates, a standard colour vision test.

Neonatal pupil

The pupil of the neonate is usually small and minimally reactive to light. The older child's pupillary size is usually larger and easily inspected.

Pupillary responses

Assessment of direct pupillary response with the swinging flashlight (afferent pupillary assessment test) may be difficult as these tests require controlling the child's fixation on a distant target rather than on the light source being used. Failure to do so will induce a near synkynesis and the resulting pupillary response will not be the consequence of light stimulation.

Ocular motor examination

Examination of the ocular motor system of children is especially important.

Strabismus

Strabismus is an extremely common disorder in children (estimated to occur in approximately 2% of non-premature infants). Assessment of ocular alignment in primary gaze is the first step in examining the ocular motor system. In the infant this may be only accomplished by examining the corneal light reflex (Hirschberg). Keeping in mind that the corneal light reflex usually appears to be just nasal to the centre of the pupil, this test can be extremely sensitive in detecting small angles of strabismus. However, the cover test and cover/uncover test are usually more accurate, especially in evaluation of small strabismic deviations. Both of these tests require controlling the child's fixation so that an accurate assessment may be obtained.

Small strabismic deviations that may not be apparent using the cover test may be detected with the 4-D base-out prism test. Introduction of the 4-D base-out prism in either eye should induce a refixation to re-establish ocular alignment if no strabismus exists. If the prism is placed in front of an eye and no refixation effort is noted, this may infer that the eye with the prism over it has a suppression scotoma due to a small strabismic deviation (Fig. 4.5). Assessment of ocular motor alignment should also be completed in the extremes of horizontal and vertical gaze. This may detect a strabismus disorder

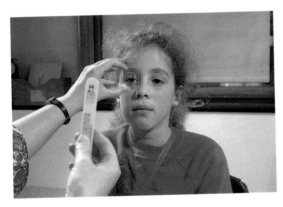

Fig. 4.5 This child is being examined with a 4-D base-out prism whilst fixation is being maintained with a hand-held acuity stick.

that is not apparent in primary gaze. This may be done by evaluation of the corneal light reflex or cover test, or alternatively by examination of ductions and versions. Overaction as well as underaction of individual extraocular muscles is important to identify. A perpetual face turn, chin position or head tilt may hide the presence of strabismus. Evaluation of ocular alignment should be carried out with the child's face in a normal, straightahead, untilted position.

Supranuclear disorders

Under certain circumstances evaluation of the supranuclear control systems may be essential. For example, poor saccadic eye movements are a common finding in the child with cerebral palsy and may be misinterpreted to imply blindness. Similarly the evaluation of nystagmus in children is a frequent clinical problem. Congenital nystagmus must be distinguished from the more ominous acquired forms. The tendency for congenital nystagmus to be made worse on fixation should be contrasted to the usual improvement seen in acquired forms of nystagmus.

Stereoacuity

The sensory consequences of strabismus may be evaluated with a number of tests. Stereopsis is a binocular function in which perception of depth perception occurs as the result of nasal or temporal disparity in the projection of visual images. Good ocular alignment as well as good visual acuity are necessary for high-grade stereoacuity to be achieved. Quantitative evaluation of stereoacuity may be assessed by the Titmus fly or Randot stereopsis test. This requires a co-operative child and failure to perform the test in young children should not be interpreted to mean that strabismus or amblyopia is necessarily present. The Randot test is usually considered to be less prone to errors as the result of monocular cues.

Fusion

Presence or absence of sensory fusion may be evaluated with the Worth four-dot test. In this test the child wears a pair of glasses with red lenses over the right eye and a green lens over the left eye. An illuminated target consisting of one red dot, two green dots and one white dot is shown to the child at various distances of fixation. The patient with normal fusion will see four dots. The patient with diplopia will report five. A patient with suppression of the right eye will report seeing three dots, whereas the patient with suppression of the left will see two. Some authorities have argued that evaluation of sensory fusion is not necessary if the careful evaluation of motor fusion has been undertaken previously.

Slit lamp examination

Slit lamp evaluation of even young children can often be undertaken successfully even without the newer hand-held slit lamps. This may be done with the child on the parent's lap or with the child kneeling in the examination chair. It is especially important in evaluating the presence or absence of conjunctival, corneal and anterior chamber pathology. It is also helpful in evaluating the child with a partial cataract in whom the decision about whether surgery is required may be especially difficult.

Intraocular pressure measurements

Although routine evaluation of intraocular pressure is not usually carried out in most children, under certain circumstances it is imperative that it be done. These include children with:

- congenital or traumatic cataracts;

- family history of early-onset glaucoma;
- systemic syndromes frequently associated with special forms of glaucoma (e.g. the Sturge–Weber syndrome);
- children on medications associated with glaucoma (e.g. steroids).

Intraocular pressure measurements may be accomplished with applanation or pneumatic techniques.

Refraction
(See Chapter 3.)

Fundus examination
Examination of the ocular fundus in infants and children may be difficult but is extremely important. Adequate mydriasis is essential and may be obtained by either cycloplegic agents alone or cycloplegic agents in conjunction with sympathomimetics. Both the indirect and direct ophthalmoscope may be useful depending on the nature of the pathology being evaluated. The increased magnification of the direct ophthalmoscope is particularly helpful in evaluating the child with a subtle optic nerve anomaly. In contrast, the indirect ophthalmoscope will be preferred in evaluating the patient with retinopathy of prematurity or other peripheral retinal diseases or disorders in which the wide-angled view is essential. The use of direct diametric-powered lenses makes the indirect ophthalmoscope more versatile. For example, a + 14-D lens provides better magnified details of the optic nerve and macular region, whereas a + 30-D lens facilitates the evaluation of the peripheral retina. Fundus photography is frequently beneficial in documenting the nature and/or change in the size of retinal lesions.

The premature infant
In most cases, examination of the premature infant is necessitated by the need to evaluate the presence or absence of retinopathy of prematurity. This requires adequate pupillary dilatation without producing iatrogenic side-effects from the agents used to accomplish it. High concentrations of sympathomimetics should be particularly avoided because of their propensity for changing the heart rate and/or blood pressure. These examinations almost always require that a lid speculum be used. An indirect ophthalmoscope with a 28- or 30-D lens is used to evaluate the retina. Indentation of the peripheral retina may be necessary in order to complete the evaluation of the entire retinal periphery. A recently completed multicentred randomised prospective trial evaluating cryotherapy in the treatment of retinopathy of prematurity has emphasised the prognostic importance of the number of clock hours of peripheral retina involved in the retinopathic process. Failure of pupillary dilatation to occur after adequate mydriatic agents have been instilled in the child with retinopathy of prematurity may occur in association with accelerated forms of retinopathy of prematurity in which an associated inflammatory process occurs.

Examination under sedation and/or anaesthesia
A standard examination may be impossible to accomplish without sedation or anaesthesia. This may be true not only in the uncooperative child but also for those requiring specific tests (e.g. electroretinography) or therapies (e.g. injection of oculinum). Sedation may be accomplished with an oral dose of chloral hydrate (50–100 mg/kg). It should be noted that in some children this will produce a paradoxical excitation and will not produce the necessary sedation. Alternatively, ketamine may be used. Under some circumstances general anaesthesia in an ambulatory surgical centre may be required in order to accomplish an extensive evaluation (e.g. a child with retinoblastoma congenital glaucoma). In many cases the examination under anaesthesia is important in determining whether or not immediate surgery may follow. Appropriate counselling of the parents is necessary in this setting so as to obviate the need for a second anaesthetic.

Systemic and developmental assessment
Photophobia
Photophobia is an abnormal sensitivity to light in an otherwise normal lighting condition, which produces discomfort, tearing, blinking or forceful closure of the eyelids as a result. Many children develop eye blinking for a period of time, with no

other signs of ocular pathology, as an apparent transient tic. The cause of photophobia may be due to pathology at several levels of the visual system including the following.

Cornea

Undoubtedly the most common site of pathology in a child with photophobia is the cornea. Pathological changes that result in disruption of the corneal epithelium or the clarity of its optical components may result in photophobia. This may occur in children with:

- congenital glaucoma;
- corneal dystrophy;
- corneal infection (especially chickenpox and measles);
- trauma;
- metabolic disturbances (e.g. tyrosinaemia type II).

The severity of photophobia associated with corneal disease may be such that pronounced epiphora accompanies it. This may be mistakenly interpreted to imply that obstruction of the nasolacrimal duct system is present.

Uvea

Disorders of the uveal tissue may be associated with photophobia. Two mechanisms are responsible for this. First, defects of the iris stroma may result in excessive light being transmitted to the retina (e.g. albinism or aniridia). Second, uveal inflammatory conditions frequently produce photophobia. This should not be interpreted to mean that all uveitic syndromes invariably are associated with photophobia. Indeed, the iritis of juvenile rheumatoid arthritis is known to be particularly sinister in its failure to produce early clinical symptoms.

Lens

Interference with the clarity of the crystalline lens may result in photophobia. Photophobia is therefore more commonly associated with partial cataracts rather than with total ones.

Vitreous

Photophobia is seen in patients with vitritis and/or metastatic endophthalmitis.

Retina

Photophobia may occur in congenital cone or cone–rod dystrophies. This is usually associated with nystagmus and reduced visual acuity. It is noteworthy that photophobia is usually not a feature of acquired cone dystrophies.

Optic nerve

Photophobia may accompany optic nerve disorders including optic neuritis and even congenital optic nerve anomalies. The mechanism whereby this occurs is not understood.

Central nervous system

Photophobia associated with central nervous system disease may be particularly apparent in acute meningitis or encephalitis, but it also may be seen in a child with cortical visual impairment of long-standing duration.

Strabismus

Photophobia and the tendency to close one eye in the bright sunlight is an almost pathognomonic feature of intermittent exotropia. It is not known to occur in esodeviations.

Eye pain

The description of ocular pain may vary from as mild a complaint as itching or scratching of the eye to severe throbbing pain associated with nausea and/or vomiting. In the younger child eye pain may be manifest by excessive eye rubbing, blinking or apparent photophobia. The pain-perceiving fibres innervating the eye and periorbital structures arise from the trigeminal or fifth cranial nerve. Different ocular structures vary in their density of pain nerve endings. For example, subepithelial corneal structures have the greatest concentration, whereas the conjunctival structures are relatively free of them. Thus, pain arising from different areas of the eye may vary in intensity. In some diseases pain perceived to arise from the eye is actually the manifestation of pathology remote to it, for example, in some forms of migraine headache.

Cornea

Undoubtedly the most common site of pathology responsible for eye pain is the cornea, particularly its subepithelial area. Thus, trauma, infection and some metabolic or dystrophic processes may produce severe eye pain.

Conjunctiva

Pure conjunctival disease is rarely associated with severe pain, although itching, scratching or a burning sensation may be reported. If severe pain accompanies conjunctival disease, associated corneal, scleral or intraocular pathology should be sought.

Sclera

Inflammation of the episclera or sclera may be associated with marked injection over the area and pain.

Tear abnormalities

Pain may occur as the result of poor tear production. This is much less common in children than in adults. In children it may occur in association with congenital syndromes (e.g. the Riley–Day syndrome), or as the result of inflammatory orbital disease (pseudotumour) or as part of a generalized host versus graft reaction.

Nasolacrimal duct obstruction

Acute dacryocystitis occurs in some infants with congenital nasolacrimal duct obstruction. The tearing associated with this may be accompanied by pain.

Glaucoma

Pain may occur in congenital or acquired glaucoma in children. It is the result of secondary corneal breakdown, particularly of the epithelium.

Iris

Many forms of iritis will present with photophobia and pain. However, some forms of iritis characteristically are silent without significant discomfort (e.g. juvenile rheumatoid arthritis). Posterior forms of uveitis primarily involving the vitreous, choroid or retina are usually not accompanied by significant pain.

Optic nerve

Isolated optic nerve or retinal disease is usually not accompanied by pain. Pain may occur in optic neuritis as the result of involvement of the inflamed nerve sheath. Optic neuritis in childhood occurs uncommonly.

Lids

Acute inflammatory disease of the lids may result in pain. This is particularly true in preseptal or septal cellulitis.

Central nervous system

Orbital or central nervous system pathology may present with eye pain. The site of the underlying pathology may involve the cavernous sinus, brainstem or third or sixth cranial nerves.

Fictitious visual pain

Although fictitious visual loss is by far the most common functional complaint, functional eye pain is not infrequent. This diagnosis cannot be established, however, until all other potential pathologies have been ruled out.

Diagnosis

Diagnosis of the cause of eye pain cannot be made until direct inspection of the eye and intraocular structures has been undertaken. Particular attention to the cornea and corneal epithelium is necessary and may require staining of the epithelium with fluorescein or rose bengal. In some cases, where eye pain is associated with severe photophobia and squeezing of the eyelids, examination under anaesthesia or sedation may be necessary to establish the appropriate diagnosis. This is especially true in the child suspected of having glaucoma, where intraocular pressure measurements are essential. Only rarely will neuroradiographical studies be necessary to evaluate the pathology outside of the eye or periorbital structures.

Treatment

Treatment of eye pain depends on establishing the underlying cause.

- Corneal abrasions: patching.
- Glaucoma: control of intraocular pressure.
- Iritis: pupillary dilatation and anti-inflammatories.

Evaluation of the child with congenital or early visual loss

A child with significant bilateral visual loss that occurs as a result of congenital or early onset pathology will usually present in two distinct ways.

Children who present with nystagmus or roving eye movements with poor visual function

This group of patients will have the cause of their visual loss within the ocular structure themselves or neural visual pathways anterior to or involving the chiasm. Thus, pathology may primarily involve the:

- cornea;
- lens;
- vitreous;
- retina;
- optic nerve;
- chiasm.

In many cases the pathology will be readily apparent on even the most perfunctory examination. For example, the child with bilateral congenital cataracts or corneal opacities will be easy to detect. This is also the case for most children in whom optic nerve dysfunction is present. Regrettably, this is not the case with most congenital retinal disorders presenting with nystagmus. Thus, most congenital cone, cone–rod and rod–cone dystrophies characteristically present with no pathological features seen on fundoscopic examination of the retina in infancy. Other findings on ophthalmic examination may be suggestive of a co-existing retinal pathology. For example:

- hypermetropia—Leber's congenital amaurosis;
- boys with myopia X-linked recessive congenital stationary night blindness and myopia or blue-cone dystrophy.

However, only appropriate electrophysiological testing with electroretinography (ERG) will be adequate to provide a specific diagnosis.

In the case of a child who presents with obvious severe optic nerve hypoplasia, no further investigation may be necessary to establish the cause of visual loss, although they may be indicated for other purposes (e.g. identifying associated central nervous system anomalies). However, in the case of a child with nystagmus and optic atrophy, neurological investigation will almost certainly be required. In this setting, hydrocephalus, optic nerve gliomas and craniopharyngiomas are the most likely cause of optic nerve atrophy.

A second group of patients who present with poor vision and no nystagmus

These children usually have:

- cortical visual impairment; or
- delayed visual maturation.

In the case of a child with cortical visual impairment, usually a history of significant perinatal problems (e.g. asphyxia) is obtained. Moreover, in most cases other signs of obvious neurological deficit are apparent: seizures, spasticity or hypotonia of the extremities. Only rarely is cortical visual impairment seen as an isolated neurological handicap. Nevertheless, the extent of the damage to the primary visual cortex and its associated areas can best be evaluated by magnetic resonance imaging (MRI) or computerized tomography (CT) scanning.

Less commonly, children who present with no apparent deficit other than poor visual function without nystagmus have no apparently cortical visual impairment. These children usually present in the first 6 months of life, and by the time they reach 1 year of age, normal visual behaviours have been noted. The term 'delayed visual maturation' has been applied to this clinical subset. Although this implies that these children have only a temporary delay in obtaining normal visual function, follow-up studies suggest that many of these children have minor associated neurological abnormalities, especially, attention disorders and minor degrees of cerebral palsy.

Acquired visual loss

Investigation of acquired visual deficit is more complex than that of the congenital one. No simple algorithmic model can be applied to this group of children. First, it is necessary to establish the site of the acquired visual deficit. Significant visual loss associated with corneal, lenticular, vitreal or retinal pathology is usually readily apparent on the appropriate ophthalmic examination. This may require slit lamp examination, direct and indirect ophthalmoscopy and, occasionally, examination under anaesthesia. In some forms of retinal disease visual loss may occur before morphological changes are apparent in the retina. Thus, in the case of Stargardt's disease no apparent defects may be noticed on ophthalmoscopy, but on fluorescein angiography a blockage of choroidal flow pattern may be seen in the early stages. Likewise, in acquired cone or cone–rod dystrophies the retina may appear grossly normal at a time when ERG testing shows it is clearly not. In the case of acquired optic nerve disease, an afferent pupillary defect or colour vision loss may be detected before significant visual acuity loss. CT or MRI scanning is frequently required in the evaluation of optic atrophy, especially when it is asymmetrical or unilateral.

5: Infectious Diseases

Prenatal infections and acquired immune deficiency syndrome (AIDS)

Rubella

Rubella infection acquired by the mother during the pregnancy, especially in early pregnancy, gives rise to a constellation of signs known as the congenital rubella syndrome (CRS).

CRS
- Eye defects:
    (a) cataracts;
    (b) retinal pigment disturbance;
    (c) glaucoma;
    (d) microphthalmos;
    (e) corneal defects;
    (f) transient corneal oedema.
- Systemic defects:
    (a) congenital heart defect;
    (b) deafness;
    (c) thrombocytopenia;
    (d) hepatosplenomegaly;
    (e) diabetes;
    (f) cerebral calcification;
    (g) microcephaly;
    (h) mental retardation.

The earlier the infection during the pregnancy the more severe the ocular and systemic damage.

Cataracts
Cataracts are bilateral in 75% of cases and are either total or consist of a shaggy central nuclear and cortical cataract. They are managed in much the same way as other causes of congenital cataract (see Chapter 14): special care needs to be taken in their management because of associated glaucoma and postoperative endophthalmitis, which can be avoided by complete lensectomy and use of topical, subconjunctival and systemic steroids (Fig. 5.1).

Pigmentary retinopathy
This is bilateral and present in the majority of affected patients. The electroretinogram is usually normal and vision is little affected by this abnormality (Fig. 5.2). Disciform degeneration may occur later.

Keratitis
Very rarely this is severe and results in scarring, but commonly there is a transient corneal haziness often mistaken for glaucoma. This usually clears spontaneously within a few days or weeks (Fig. 5.3).

Glaucoma
This may occur in approximately 10% of children with CRS. Initially, treatment may be with acetazolamide and antiglaucoma drops, but the definitive treatment is surgery (see Chapter 15). Beta-blocker drops should be used with care in those children who may have lung and heart disorders.

Iris hypoplasia
This usually has few functional effects but may indicate severe intraocular damage.

CRS is seen much less frequently now that rubella vaccination is widespread.

Diagnosis
The diagnosis is usually suspected on the history of a rash and fever in pregnancy, or the finding of signs compatible with CRS. Virus may be isolated from the urine, saliva or lens aspirate (for up to 4 years). Rubella-specific immunoglobulin M (IgM) persists in infants with CRS.

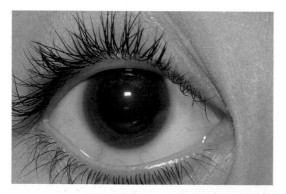

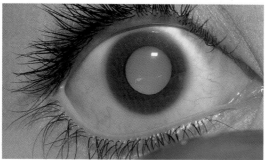

Fig. 5.1 Congenital rubella cataract. Twenty-five per cent have a unilateral cataract associated with microphthalmos. Virus can be grown from the lens up to 4 years of age.

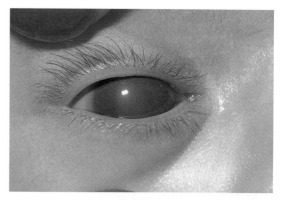

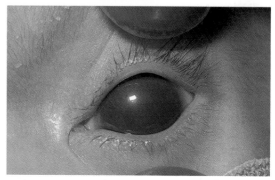

Fig. 5.3 Neonate with congenital rubella with hazy large appearing corneas. The intraocular pressures were normal.

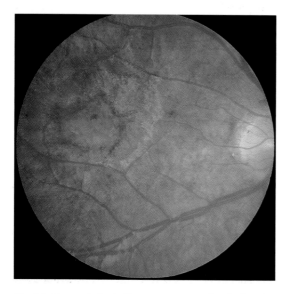

Fig. 5.2 Congenital rubella retinopathy. There are diffuse retinal pigment epithelial changes most marked at the posterior pole. The acuity is 6/12.

Management

Cataracts are usually treated early with lensectomy covered with steroids. In the management of glaucoma it is important to exclude rubella keratopathy as the cause of the cloudy cornea. Careful intraocular pressure measurement is mandatory. The management of the baby with CRS requires a multidisciplinary approach.

Toxoplasmosis

The incidence of toxoplasmosis varies widely throughout the world, some areas having a very high incidence whereas in others it is of little significance. After birth it causes a febrile illness and lymphadenopathy of little consequence, unless it affects a pregnant woman when the fetus may be variably affected. Infection early in the first trimester, especially if severe, may cause fetal death; later and less severe infections cause less severe disease. Only a small proportion of infected mothers have affected babies.

- The congenital toxoplasmosis syndrome (CTS) includes:
  (a) intracranial calcification;
  (b) hydrocephalus;
  (c) microcephaly;
  (d) seizures;
  (e) hepatitis;
  (f) fever;
  (g) anaemia;
  (h) deafness;
  (i) mental retardation.
- Ocular manifestations of CTS include:
  (a) chorioretinitis;
  (b) uveitis;
  (c) cerebral blindness;
  (d) cataract (secondary to uveitis).

Chorioretinitis

Chorioretinitis is the most common manifestation of CTS. It is usually focal with areas of chorioretinal atrophy and hyperpigmentation. It is usually bilateral and mostly affects the posterior pole (Fig. 5.4). Reactivation of the uveitis may occur at any time during the child's subsequent life.

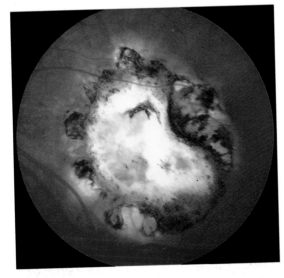

Fig. 5.4 Raised toxoplasmosis macular scar.

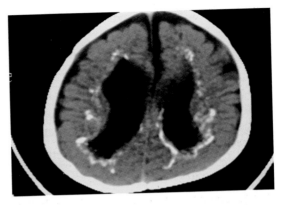

Fig. 5.5 Congenital CMV infection with periventricular calcification, hydrocephalus and cerebral atrophy shown on this CT scan.

Other ocular abnormalities

Microphthalmos, cataracts and panuveitis may occur in more severely affected patients. The cataracts are usually the non-specific result of intraocular inflammation and are nearly always accompanied by very severe retinal disease. Optic atrophy may occur as a result of hydrocephalus or a severely affected brain (Fig. 5.5).

Diagnosis

Diagnosis is usually by serology; cultures are rarely used. The Dye test depends on the inhibition of live *Toxoplasma gondii* by antibodies in the patient's serum. Dye titres rise in acute infections, but the infant's serum may contain passively transferred antibody, so a rising titre must be demonstrated, or an enzyme-linked immunosorbent assay (ELISA) test for IgM must be positive.

Management

Affected neonates who are seropositive, having anti-*Toxoplasma* IgM, are treated with pyrimethamine (1 mg/kg per day) and sulphadiazine (100 mg/kg per day) for 10–21 days together with folinic acid. Pregnant women with primary toxoplasmosis infection may be treated with spiramycin but should not be treated with pyrimethamine and sulphadiazine.

Screening for toxoplasmosis is still controversial and policies vary in different countries.

Patients with cataracts should be investigated with ultrasound, visual evoked potentials and electroretinography to see if they have good retinal function and visual potential. Acute exacerbations of chorioretinitis should be treated with systemic steroids and pyrimethamine/folinic acid/sulphadiazimine or with spiramycin. This is usually best carried out under the care of a paediatric infective diseases expert.

Cytomegalovirus (CMV)

CMV infection in the newborn is very common, occurring in up to 2.5% of all newborn children. Only a few have serious problems.

- Congenital CMV systemic abnormalities:
  (a) hepatopathy;
  (b) jaundice;
  (c) pneumonitis;
  (d) microcephaly;
  (e) brain calcification;
  (f) mental retardation;
  (g) deafness;
  (h) skin rashes;
  (i) bone lesions.
- Ocular manifestations of congenital CMV:
  (a) chorioretinitis;
  (b) microphthalmos;
  (c) keratitis;
  (d) cataracts;
  (e) optic atrophy.

Eye damage in CMV infections in neonates is fortunately rare. Chorioretinitis is probably the most common and sometimes a keratitis occurs with scarring. Cataracts and microphthalmos usually occur in severely affected eyes with other blinding abnormalities.

Herpes simplex

Neonatal herpes simplex occurs in children whose mother's have genital herpes simplex infection. The infection is nearly always symptomatic and is transmitted during birth or, rarely, *in utero*, after rupture of the membranes. Systemic infection carries a high morbidity and mortality.

- Herpes simplex systemic involvement:
  (a) skin rash in nearly 100%;
  (b) hepatitis;
  (c) pneumonitis;
  (d) encephalitis.
- Ocular involvement in neonatal herpes simplex:
  (a) acute conjunctivitis and blepharitis with lid vesicles;
  (b) chorioretinitis;
  (c) uveitis;
  (d) rarely, necrotizing uveitis;
  (e) cataracts.

The most severe eye damage from herpes simplex is usually to the cornea with an acute keratoconjunctivitis, sometimes with epithelial dendrites and a stromal keratitis. A peripheral retinitis is much less frequent.

Diagnosis

The diagnosis is made either by scraping the vesicles which are then looked at for the presence of multinucleated giant cells, by culture of the vesicles or by way of IgM-specific antiherpes antibodies.

Management

Systemic treatment with acyclovir (30 mg/kg per day in three divided doses intravenously) is often used for the systemic manifestations.

Herpes keratoconjunctivitis should be treated either with idoxuridine, acyclovir or triflurothymidine topically.

Congenital syphilis

Congenital syphilis may be increasing in certain social subgroups, and it has important eye manifestations. Infection before 18 weeks of gestation probably has little effect on the fetus; after that time infection and fetal damage may occur, especially in severe and untreated maternal infections.

- Systemic manifestations include:
  (a) maculopapular rash;
  (b) rhinitis;
  (c) skeletal abnormalities;
  (d) nose fissures;
  (e) hepatopathy;
  (f) anaemia;
  (g) uveitis;
  (h) deafness;
  (i) dental abnormalities.

- Eye abnormalities in congenital syphilis include:
    (a) chorioretinitis;
    (b) uveitis;
    (c) interstitial keratitis;
    (d) optic atrophy.

Interstitial keratitis is the most common eye manifestation of congenital syphilis. It is usually bilateral and sectorial with oedema and vascularization (the so-called 'salmon patch'). Chorioretinitis is less common.

The diagnosis requires a venereal disease reference test (VDRT) that is higher in the baby than its mother. It is usually treated with a prolonged course of systemic penicillin.

Congenital varicella

Although a rare cause of pre-natal eye and brain damage, varicella may cause severe, and often overlooked, problems. Infection early in pregnancy usually causes fetal death or severe congenital manifestations; these may be prevented by hyperimmune globulin. Maternal infection around birth may give rise to varicella or zoster-type skin lesions in the infant, which may be prevented by hyperimmune globulin.

- Systemic manifestations include:
    (a) skin scarring;
    (b) cerebral damage;
    (c) seizures;
    (d) limb malformations.

- Congenital varicella eye manifestations include:
    (a) chorioretinitis;
    (b) cataracts;
    (c) Horner's syndrome;
    (d) microphthalmos;
    (e) uveitis.

Chorioretinitis is the most common ocular manifestation of congenital varicella. It is similar to the chorioretinitis of congenital toxoplasmosis. The scars are multiple, and often bilateral. Severe intraocular damage may result in cataracts and microphthalmos. Neurological damage manifests itself as optic atrophy, Horner's syndrome and brain blindness including hemianopias (Fig. 5.6).

Management consists of serological diagnosis and the treatment of pregnant women exposed to varicella and perinatally infected women and children with immune globulin. Only the skin lesions usually benefit from treatment; immune compromised children with varicella may require systemic acyclovir or gancyclovir.

Congenital human immunodeficiency virus (HIV) infection

This occurs by transplacental transmission of HIV from an infected mother; the prevalence in infants born to infected women is up to 40%. It can also occur peri-natally. Post-natal infection occurs by the use of infected blood products, and in adolescents or abused children by sexual contact with an infected person.

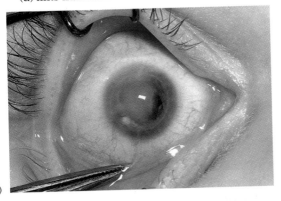
(a)

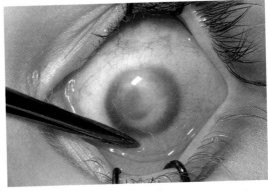
(b)

Fig. 5.6 Congenital rubella with microphthalmos cataract, iris damage glaucoma, and corneal scaring. The right eye (a) had had a partially successful graft and had navigation vision.

- Systemic manifestations include:
  (a) opportunistic infections;
  (b) pneumonitis;
  (c) encephalitis;
  (d) failure to thrive.
- Eye manifestations include:
  (a) HIV retinopathy;
  (b) opportunistic infections;
  (c) CMV retinitis, toxoplasmosis;
  (d) retinal necrosis;
  (e) adnexal disease.

HIV retinopathy

HIV retinopathy is of unknown cause and consists of cotton wool spots and retinal haemorrhages with other vascular changes.

Opportunistic infections: CMV retinitis

This is the most common manifestation of immune deficiency. The initial lesions are cotton wool spots with haemorrhages, usually with central necrosis. The lesions spread out from the originally affected area and satellites occur. Treatment is with gancyclovir or foscarnet via a long intravenous line. Cure is rarely achieved.

Toxoplasmosis

Toxoplasmosis occurs as a severe rapid necrotizing retinochoroiditis and uveitis. It is treated with sulphadiazine and pyrimethamine, but relapse is frequent.

Retinal necrosis

This presents as a necrotic pale swollen retina with separate lesions becoming confluent. It may be due to herpes zoster or herpes simplex.

Adnexal disease

Conjunctival Kaposi's sarcoma, large molluscum contagiosum lesions and herpes simplex keratitis may sometimes also occur.

Diagnosis

Diagnosis of neonatal HIV infection can be difficult. HIV can be cultured, or HIV deoxyribonucleic acid (DNA) detected by polymerized chain reaction or HIV P24 antigen can be detected in the infant's serum.

Conjunctivitis and the newborn

Chlamydial conjunctivitis

Chlamydia trachomatis is the most common cause of neonatal conjunctivitis in the West. It is unilateral, becoming bilateral and associated with pneumonitis. The lids are swollen and there is a watery discharge with some mucus and mucopus. Treatment is with a short course of erythromycin syrup, 40 mg/kg per day for 14 days. The parents should be treated as well. Oral treatment is more effective than topical treatment (Fig. 5.7).

Gonococcal conjunctivitis

This presents in the first few days of life with a rapidly progressive severe purulent conjunctivitis. The cornea is rapidly affected. Treatment is either with penicillin (benzylpenicillin 30 mg/kg per day in two or three divided doses) or, when penicillinase-producing *Neisseria gonorrhoeae* (PPNG) are present, a cephalosporin (such as cephuroxime 100 mg/kg per day in three divided doses for 7 days) may be used. Topical antibiotics such as erythromycin 1%, or gentamycin 1% can also be used for PPNG. Frequent irrigation of the eye with warm normal saline is sometimes recommended.

Other organisms include: *Staphylococcus aureus, Staph. epidermidis, Streptococcus viridans, Strep. pneumoniae, Escherichia coli, Serratia* spp., *Pseudomonas* spp. and *Haemophilus* spp.

Box 5.1 The sticky eye in childhood

1 Nasolacrimal duct obstruction:
  (a) with mucocoele;
  (b) without mucocoele (usually associated with epiphora).
2 Conjunctivitis:
  (a) in the neonate;
  (b) in infancy and childhood—bacterial, viral or other.
3 Allergic conjunctivitis: associated with itching, lid oedema and a mucopurulent discharge.
4 Vernal conjunctivitis with keratitis and giant lid papillae.
5 Cat scratch disease.
6 Dry eye.
7 Foreign bodies.

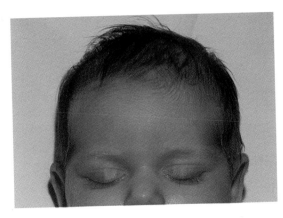

Fig. 5.7 Neonatal chlamydial conjunctivitis. The lids are swollen and there is a discharge.

Viral conjunctivitis

Viral conjunctivitis can be caused by herpes simplex virus. Occasionally, adenovirus infections occur in the first few days of life and need to be treated appropriately.

Investigation

Clinical investigation is most important. It is vital to be sure that the child does not have a congenital nasolacrimal duct obstruction. This can be diagnosed by the history or by refluxing mucopurulent material with pressure over the lacrimal sac. A Gram's stain of a conjunctival scrape should be performed looking for Gram-negative diplococci in particular, or other bacterial species. *Chlamydia* can be diagnosed by McCoy cell culture or by polymerised chain reaction. A Giemsa's stain may identify intracytoplasmic inclusion bodies of *Chlamydia*. Bacterial and viral cultures need to be carried out for the other organisms.

Prophylaxis

Prophylaxis with silver nitrate 1% is now rarely used. There is no world-wide policy but the following are used:
- topical erythromycin 0.5% ointment;
- topical tetracycline 1% ointment;
- povidone–iodine.

Orbital and preseptal cellulitis

Preseptal cellulitis

Preseptal cellulitis occurs when an orbital infection is limited to being anterior to the orbital septum which prevents spread to the orbit itself (Fig. 5.8).

Aetiology

1 Lid infections, i.e. herpes simplex, acute blepharitis, infected chalazion, impetigo and skin abscess.
2 Dacryocystitis.
3 Trauma with suppurative cellulitis, *Staph. aureus* and beta-haemolytic *Streptococcus*.
4 Upper respiratory tract infection, *Haemophilus influenzae* and *Streptococcus*. *H. influenzae* infections most frequently occur in very young children.

Clinical presentation

The child usually presents with unilateral lid oedema, fever with a leucocytosis and local abnormalities may be found, i.e. chalazion, dacryocystitis, etc. Discharge and watering may occur.

Management

Diagnosis
- Gram's stain of any discharge.
- Blood culture and culture of any discharge.
- Plain X-rays or a computerized tomography (CT) scan for associated sinus disease.

Treatment
Most patients are treated as in-patients, preferably

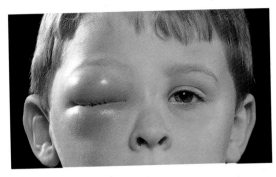

Fig. 5.8 Preseptal cellulitis associated with sinusitis in an otherwise healthy child.

jointly by a paediatrician and/or infectious diseases consultant.

Antibiotic treatment

If there are clear indications on the Gram's stain, treatment specific to the likely organism is given pending the results of the culture and sensitivity. It is important not to start treatment before the cultures have been taken, including blood cultures.

When associated with trauma, oxacillin or nafcillin 150–200 mg/kg per day is used; when associated with an upper respiratory tract infection, cefuroxime 100–150 mg/kg per day or a combination of ampicillin 50–100 mg/kg per day with chloramphenicol 75–100 mg/kg per day are used. Chloramphenicol is not available in some countries due to concern about side-effects. At least initially, intravenous treatment is given. When the local and blood cultures are returned, if there is not already a good clinical improvement, the antibiotic can be changed appropriately.

Surgical drainage of an abscess is rarely necessary, it is performed when the abscess shows no signs of resolving after several days of antibody treatment.

Orbital cellulitis

Orbital cellulitis occurs when the infection is behind the orbital septum; it may be associated with preseptal cellulitis.

Aetiology

1 Trauma.
2 Foreign body.
3 Post-surgical.
4 Haematogeneous, i.e. during a systemic infectious disease.
5 Secondary to a necrotic neoblastoma.
6 Associated with sinus disease.

Causative organisms

1 *H. influenzae* in infants.
2 *Staph. aureus*.
3 *Strep. pyogenes* and *Strep. pneumoniae*.
4 *E. coli*.
5 Fungi and mucor (in immunosuppressed or diabetic children).

Presentation

1 Proptosis.
2 Pain.
3 Lid oedema.
4 Poor vision.
5 Chemosis.
6 Limited eye movement.
7 Fever and systemic illness.
8 Optic neuropathy leading to optic atrophy.
9 Keratitis from exposure due to proptosis.
10 Central retinal artery occlusion.
11 Subperiosteal abscess, associated with sinus disease (Fig. 5.9).
12 Orbital abscess.
13 Cavernous sinus thrombosis.
14 Meningitis.
15 Brain abscess.
16 Septicaemia.

Management

The patient is always admitted to hospital.

Investigations

1 For Gram's stain culture and sensitivity to antibiotics, take swabs of:
  (a) conjunctiva; and
  (b) nose/throat.

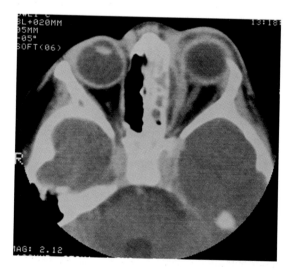

Fig. 5.9 CT scan showing left ethmoidal sinusitis and subperiosteal abscess.

2 Sinus X-rays.

3 CT scan to assess the extent of orbital involvement, to look for orbital and subperiosteal abscess formation.

4 Ear, nose and throat consultation.

5 Dental examination if necessary.

6 Search for remote septic foci.

7 Lumbar puncture if meningitis suspected.

8 Blood culture.

Management is preferably carried out in conjunction with a paediatrician and infectious diseases consultant.

Treatment

1 Where initial Gram's stains point to a specific organism, the antibiotic treatment is directed towards that specific organism pending the results of the other tests.

2 Where no particular organism is suspected the treatment may be:

(a) intravenous chloramphenicol (75–100 mg/kg per day) combined with intravenous ampicillin (150 mg/kg per day);

(b) a cephalosporin, i.e. ceftazidime 100–150 mg/kg per day, ceftriaxone 100–150 mg/kg per day combined with nafcillin or oxacillin 150–200 mg/kg per day.

Drainage of an abscess may be necessary.

It is important not to discharge the child until he/she is completely well, and to carry on the antibiotics for at least 1 week after the improvement of the fever and the beginning of resolution of the condition. Failure to do this or treating with an inadequate dose may result in relapse, osteomyelitis and other complications.

It is important to watch for the occurrence of complications even if the clinical appearance is improving, i.e. pupil reactions may suggest an optic neuropathy or retinal vascular disease, and if proptosis does not resolve serial CT scans may be necessary.

Endophthalmitis

Endophthalmitis occurs when the inner contents of the eye are infected. Panophthalmitis is a term used when the infection is widespread, affecting all parts of the eye. It may be difficult to diagnose endophthalmitis in children because of the difficulty in examination, but the following features are usually present:

1 predisposing cause, i.e. trauma, surgery, etc.;

2 lid swelling;

3 conjunctival injection and chemosis;

4 uveitis;

5 hypopion;

6 retinal vascular dilatation.

The severity and rapidity of the onset of the endophthalmitis depends on the route of entry and with the organism. For instance, *Streptococcus* spp. and *Pseudomonas* tend to give rapidly progressive severely damaging endophthalmitis. *Staphylococcus* spp., especially *Staph. epidermidis*, give milder signs, the onset of which may be delayed. Fungal endophthalmitis is usually less severe but not necessarily less damaging.

Aetiology

1 Trauma—surgical—penetrating trauma.

2 Keratitis: if the infective organisms penetrate Descemet's membrane an infective anterior uveitis and, ultimately, endophthalmitis may occur.

3 Metastatic endophthalmitis, i.e. from meningitis (especially meningococcus), bacterial endocarditis, systemic infections including otitis media. Many of these cases are often bilateral and often late diagnosed because of the overwhelming nature of the systemic infection (Fig. 5.10).

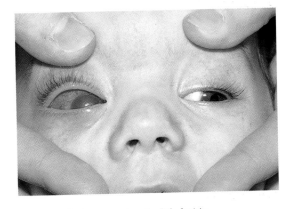

Fig. 5.10 Meningococcal endophthalmitis.

Infecting agents

Bacterial

Streptococcus and *Staphylococcus* spp. are the most frequent, especially after surgery. *Proteus* and *Pseudomonas*, often mixed with other bacteria occur after trauma. *Pseudomonas* keratitis often develops into endophthalmitis (Fig. 5.11).

Fungi

Candida spp. infection is usually associated with immune deficiency or in otherwise severely ill children. Other fungi may be involved in penetrating trauma.

Investigation

1 Gram's stain of smear.
2 Giemsa's stain of smear (especially for fungi).
3 Blood culture.
4 Anterior chamber and/or vitreous tap for smear and culture.

The specimens should be plated immediately onto blood agar, thioglycolate and chocolate agar plates, and fungi are looked for by culture in Sabouraud's medium and blood agar.

Ultrasound studies may be necessary to investigate the involvement of the posterior segment in predominantly anterior segment disease. Systemic investigations may need to be carried out for metastatic endophthalmitis.

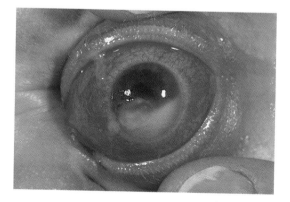

Fig. 5.11 Endophthalmitis and hypopyon following exposure keratitis. Although the eye was saved by prompt antibiotic treatment, the acuity 5 years later was very poor due to amblyopia.

Treatment

Antibiotic therapy

Bacterial endophthalmitis. Specific antibiotic treatment can be given based on the results of the various cultures and smears. If no results are forthcoming the following regimen may be used.
1 Topical:
  (a) hourly gentamicin drops (preferably without preservatives);
  (b) cephuroxime 5% drops hourly (preferably without preservative);
  (c) atropine 1% drops twice a day (0.5% twice a day in infants).
2 Subconjunctival injection (usually carried out at the same time as a vitreous tap):
  (a) gentamicin 40 mg;
  (b) cephazoline 125 mg.
3 Intravitreous injections:
  (a) gentamicin 0.1 mg in 0.1 ml;
  (b) ceftazidime 2.25 mg in 0.1 ml.
4 Systemic antibiotics:
  (a) gentamicin 2 mg/kg per day intravenously;
  (b) cefuroxrime 60 mg/kg per day in divided doses intravenously.

Fungal endophthalmitis. *Candida* is usually treated with ketoconazole or amphotericin B with flucytosine. Most other fungi are treated with amphotericin B which may be given intravitreally (5 μg).

Vitrectomy

In some cases, there may be a role for early vitrectomy to remove a large proportion of the infecting agent, to remove any foreign bodies or necrotic material and at the same time to inject antibiotics intravitreally and subconjunctivally.

Other forms of endophthalmitis

Toxocara and toxoplasmosis may occasionally present with an endophthalmitis-like appearance. In Behçet's disease the uveitis may be so severe as to mimic endophthalmitis.

Infectious conjunctivitis

Conjunctivitis is diagnosed clinically on the basis of the following findings:

1 mucopurulent discharge;
2 redness of the conjunctiva sometimes accompanied by haemorrhages and swelling;
3 watering of the eye;
4 a sensation of hotness of the eye;
5 itching is a minor and usually not very significant symptom;
6 vision is unaffected except by mucus;
7 a gritty sensation sometimes occurs if there is an associated keratitis.

Diagnosis
1 By history, taking particular note of the discharge and the presence of any systemic illness, sore throat, etc.
2 Examination:
   (a) acuity should be normal unless there is an associated keratitis or mucus production;
   (b) slit lamp examination will show conjunctival changes and sometimes the presence of an associated keratitis;
   (c) skin rashes must be looked for and the throat and lymph glands examined.
3 Laboratory diagnosis. This is not usually necessary in a primary care setting or by most general paediatricians or ophthalmologists. Conjunctivitis is so common, and usually due to virus infections that are effectively untreatable or bacterial infections that respond easily to antibiotics, that culture is not usually necessary. Culture is reserved for severe cases in chronic or recurrent infections (after stopping antibiotic treatment) and in follicular conjunctivitis or an atypical reaction.

Acute catarrhal conjunctivitis
Clinical features
1 Conjunctival injection, redness.
2 Watering.
3 Discharge.

Organisms
1 *H. influenzae.*
2 *Strep. pneumoniae.*
3 *Moraxella* (external angular conjunctivitis).
4 *Neisseria* spp.
5 *Chlamydia* in older children and adolescents.

Acute follicular conjunctivitis
Epidemic keratoconjunctivitis (EKC)
EKC is a highly infectious conjunctivitis associated with a red and watering eye, a mild keratitis (with small white epithelial and subepithelial lesions in the periphery of the cornea), sometimes with a fever. There are numerous follicles in the fornices. The main infectious agent is adenovirus. Treatment is not usually helpful but dilute steroids may improve the symptoms; the patient should be watched carefully. Antibiotic treatment may be used to prevent secondary bacterial infection.

Pharyngoconjunctival fever
Pharyngoconjunctival fever is another highly infectious keratoconjunctivitis, usually adenovirus, which is accompanied by a fever, pharyngitis and a lympadenopathy.

Herpes simplex keratoconjunctivitis
Herpes simplex keratoconjunctivitis usually occurs in older children but occasionally it occurs in neonates and young children.
   Symptoms are of redness, watering, discharge, itching, pre-auricular lymphadenopathy and the signs are of lid vesicles, lid rash, capillary conjunctivitis, punctate epithelial keratitis, dendritic keratitis, disciform keratitis and stromal keratitis.
   Treatment is with idoxuridine or acyclovir ointment. Special precautions need to be taken in the immune compromised child.

Haemorrhagic conjunctivitis
Symptoms are of redness, watering, grittiness and multiple subconjunctival haemorrhages. Picornavirus or Coxsackie virus are the usual infectious agents and the infection usually lasts just a few days and does not require treatment.

Acute conjunctivitis with systemic disease
1 *Chlamydia.*
2 Varicella.
3 Lyme Borreliosis.
4 Influenza.
5 Epstein–Barr.
6 Parinaud's oculoglandular syndrome (conjunctivitis and lymphadenopathy).

7 Sweet's syndrome: fever, arthritis and pseudovesicular skin rash.

Membranous conjunctivitis

Membranous conjunctivitis is diagnosed when the conjunctiva is covered with a fibrinous membrane on the cornea. It is seen with:

1 Stevens–Johnson syndrome;
2 toxic epidermal necrolysis;
3 herpes simplex;
4 herpes zoster;
5 *Corynebacterium diphtheriae*;
6 *Strep. pyogenes*;
7 *Staph. aureus*;
8 *Neisseria* spp.;
9 *Shigella*;
10 *Salmonella*;
11 *E. coli*.

Normal childhood folliculosis

Many children have follicles in the fornices which cause no problem. This is known as folliculosis (Fig. 5.12).

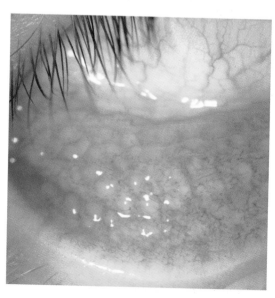

Fig. 5.12 Acute follicular conjunctivitis in a child with multiple molluscum contagiosum lesions.

Subacute and chronic follicular conjunctivitis

1 *Moraxella* external angular conjunctivitis.
2 Molluscum contagiosum.
3 Tuberous conjunctivitis.
4 Drugs: topical, especially those with preservatives may cause a chronic conjunctivitis.
5 Rosacea occurs rarely in young children.
6 Blepharoconjunctivitis.

Investigation

Where appropriate, investigation consists of conjunctival and, occasionally, scrapes for Gram's and Giemsa's stain and culture and sensitivity. Fungal and viral culture are also important as clinically directed.

Treatment

When the diagnosis can be made on bacteriological or other grounds the treatment is specific to the condition. Acute follicular conjunctivitis is usually managed symptomatically or with tobramycin or chloramphenicol to prevent secondary bacterial infection. *Chlamydia* is treated with tetracycline or erthryomycin, and molluscum contagiosum by curettage.

Catarrhal conjunctivitis

If no bacteriological diagnosis is possible then treatment with gentamicin, tobramycin or chloramphenicol in the first instance is useful until the bacteriological results have returned. If a clinical improvement is being made the original treatment is continued, even if the antibiotic sensitivities indicate that the organism is not sensitive to the antibiotic being used.

Keratitis

Interstitial keratitis

- Syphilis: see pre-natal infection.
- Other causes:
    (a) leprosy;
    (b) tuberculosis;
    (c) onchocerciasis;
    (d) herpes simplex;
    (e) measles.

Nummular keratitis

- Small multiple anterior stromal corneal lesions:
  (a) adenovirus (Fig. 5.13);
  (b) herpes simplex;
  (c) varicella–zoster;
  (d) Epstein–Barr;
  (e) sarcoid;
  (f) onchocerciasis.

Bacterial keratitis

Predisposing factors

- Trauma.
- Surgery.
- Immune deficiency.
- Exposure.
- Dry eye.
- Contact lens wear.
- Severe systemic disease.
- Trichiasis.
- Ionizing radiation—dry eye.
- Topical steroid use.
- Corneal toxic drugs.

Infecting organisms

Certain clinical clues may point to the infecting organism.

1 *Pseudomonas* corneal ulcers are rapidly advancing and liquefying; they most frequently occur in young children and contact lens wearers (Fig. 5.14).

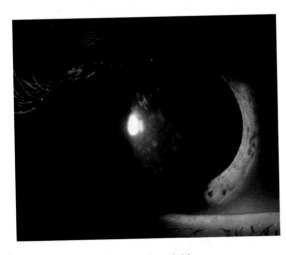

Fig. 5.13 Epidemic keratoconjunctivitis.

Box 5.2 The red eye in infancy

1 Conjunctivitis:
   (a) discharge, redness;
   (b) watering, vision normal.
2 Keratitis:
   (a) redness, discomfort, watering:
   (b) discharge, photophobia.
3 Endophthalmitis:
   (a) pain, poor vision, redness;
   (b) watering, discharge.
4 Uveitis:
   (a) pain, photophobia, blurred vision;
   (b) redness, watering.
5 Chorioretinitis:
   (a) poor vision, floaters, redness;
   (b) subconjunctival haemorrhage, redness.
6 Glaucoma:
   (a) pain, redness;
   (b) photophobia, poor vision.
7 Conjunctival infiltration—leukaemia:
   (a) localized swelling;
   (b) redness.
8 Vascular malformations:
   (a) i.e. Sturge–Weber syndrome;
   (b) orbital vascular malformation.
9 Scleritis:
   (a) pain, deep redness;
   (b) pain on movement,.
10 Episcleritis:
   (a) localized conjunctival and subconjunctival redness;
   (b) watering, mild discomfort, dry eye, redness, minimal discharge.
11 Foreign body:
   (a) localized redness, grittiness;
   (b) foreign body sensation.
12 Trauma:
   (a) direct trauma;
   (b) closed head trauma giving carotid–cavernous fistula.

---

2 *Moraxella*: associated with external angular conjunctivitis.
3 *Staphylococcus* spp.:
   (a) trauma, surgery or exposure;
   (b) *Staph. aureus* may cause a hypopion ulcer.
4 *Streptococcus*:
   (a) contact lens wearers;
   (b) locally compromised corneas;
   (c) chronic dacryocystitis;

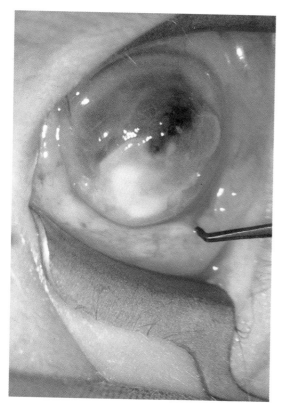

Fig. 5.14 *Pseudomonas* keratitis in a neonate with no known predisposing factors.

(d) rapidly progressing ulcers with an under-mined edge.

5 *Gonococcus*: see 'Conjunctivitis and the newborn', p. 28.

6 Gram-negative bacteria:

  (a) *E. coli*;

  (b) *Aerobacter*;

  (c) *Proteus* spp.;

  (d) *Klebsiella* spp.

These usually affect locally and systemically com-promised cornea.

Diagnosis and treatment

The diagnosis is usually made by microscopy and culture of swabs or corneal scrapings. If the patient is on treatment, it may be helpful to stop it for 24 hours before re-starting antibiotics.

Any necrotic material should be debrided and contact lenses should be removed. Local factors such as exposure must be remedied. Some small and frightened children need sedation and all need skilled nursing care.

Until antibiotic sensitivities are obtained, it is best to start treatment with hourly or half-hourly antibi-otic drops, preferably without preservatives which may be corneotoxic. Chloromycetin, gentamycin or cephalosporin drops may be used.

Virus keratitis

Herpes simplex

Punctate lesions occur most commonly and they may develop into dendrites in acute primary herpes simplex infections, which are usually associated with skin lesions. It is treated with antiviral agents, such as idoxuridine, triflurothymidine or acyclovir.

Deep non-suppurative (disciform) keratitis may occur. It may be treated with a combination of antiviral agents and steroids.

Other causes of viral keratitis include adenovirus, molloscum contagiosum, papillomas and verrucas, and Epstein–Barr virus.

Fungus keratitis

Fungus keratitis occurs in locally and systemically compromised children, i.e. those on systemic

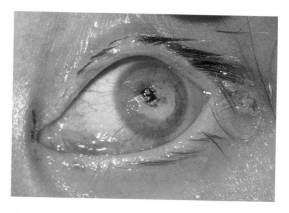

Fig. 5.15 Bilateral *Candida* keratitis in a severely immunocompromised child.

steroids, immunosuppressives, or those with trauma, dry eyes and poorly healing wounds.

Causative organisms
- *Actinomyces.*
- *Candida* (Fig. 5.15).
- *Nocardia.*
- *Fusarium.*
- Mucor.

The ulcers are usually liquefactive, slowly progressive, resistant to antibiotic treatment and may have satellite lesions.

Protozoal keratitis

Acanthamoeba keratitis occurs in contact lens users and people who swim in brackish water. *Acanthamoeba* produces chronic indolent ulcers and stromal infiltrates together with an anterior uveitis. Treatment with 0.1% propamidine isesthionate, 0.15% dibromopropamidine, neomycin or miconazole has sometimes been successful.

6: Non-infectious External Eye Disease

Allergic eye disease

All forms of allergic eye disease have certain symptoms in common.

1 Itching. This is the most prominent and constant feature present in all forms.

2 Redness.

3 Mucoid discharge.

Seasonal allergic (hayfever) conjunctivitis

- Recurrent, seasonal red eyes.
- Running nose.
- Defined allergens (pollen, etc.).
- Rapid onset.
- Itching.
- Swollen lids.
- Chemosis.
- Red eye, mucoid discharge.
- Family history.

Chronic atrophic conjunctivitis and keratoconjunctivitis

- Itching.
- Redness.
- Burning.
- Watering.
- Mucoid discharge.
- Older children.
- Often associated with eczema.
- Keratitis.

Treatment
- Decongestants.
- Antihistamine drops.
- Systemic antihistamines.
- Sodium chromoglycate drops or ointment.
- Lodoxamide.
- Cold compresses for acute attacks.

Vernal conjunctivitis

- Usually seasonal onset, becomes perennial.
- Onset after 4 years.
- Other hypersensitivity phenomena present.
- Symptoms:
  (a) redness;
  (b) itching;
  (c) watering;
  (d) lid swelling;
  (e) mucoid discharge.

Palpebral vernal conjunctivitis
- Bulbar and palpebral injection, few follicles.
- Large 'juicy' giant papillae (Fig. 6.1).

Most vernal keratitis starts in the upper third of the cornea as punctate epithelial opacities which coalesce to give macular erosion. Subepithelial scarring follows. Corneal epithelial erosions may coalesce, fill with mucus, fibrin and cells. This is vernal 'plaque'.

Limbal vernal conjunctivitis
- Swelling and opacification of the limbus with white deposits (Trantas' spots) (Fig. 6.2).
- Subepithelial limbal, vascularization, arcus lipoides.

Treatment
Acute and severe disease. Soluble steroids, i.e. fluorometholone, prednisolone, etc., by drop and ointment. These should not be used for more than 1 month unless the child is under close ophthalmological supervision, including tonometry. Disodium cromoglycate or lodoxamide can be used three to five times a day in drop form or ointment at night. It may take some days to become effective.

Decongestants and antihistamines may play some role. Vernal plaque may need to be removed surgically but it requires concurrent medical treat-

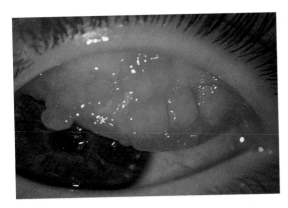

Fig. 6.1 Giant papillae in active vernal disease.

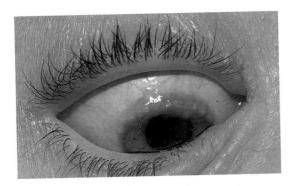

Fig. 6.2 Limbal vernal showing Trantas' spots.

ment. Giant papillae usually respond to medical treatment. Acute symptoms may be helped by cold compresses.

In chronic vernal it is best to avoid the use of steroids.

Physical and chemical irritants including many topical drugs and contact lenses

Industrial and other chemicals may give rise to a chronic papillary conjunctivitis. Acute conjunctivitis in a contact lens wearer should always be treated with suspicion, as hypoxic ulcers and quickly progressing bacterial ulcers are not infrequent. The lenses may be ill-fitting or the patient may have developed a chronic papillary conjunctival reaction to them.

Conjunctivitis artefacta

Conjunctivitis artefacta or self-inflicted conjunctivitis by burning or chemical irritants usually occurs in the lower third of the bulbar and lower palpebral conjunctiva and is associated often with lid and cheek irritation.

Phlyctenular disease

Phlyctenular conjunctivitis may be associated with tuberculosis or staphylococcal lid disease, but is usually idiopathic:
- a single localized inflammatory lesion with a white centre adjacent to the limbus;
- transient;
- lasts up to 2 weeks;
- recurrent;
- few symptoms.

Ligneous conjunctivitis

- Thickened nodular 'woody masses' in the conjunctiva.
- Cause generally unknown, sometimes after surgery or infection, occasionally autosomal recessive.
- Recurs after excision, spontaneous resolution occurs.

Biotinidase deficiency

- Conjunctivitis.
- Hypotonia.
- Seizures.
- Alopecia.
- Optic atrophy.
- Treated with biotin.

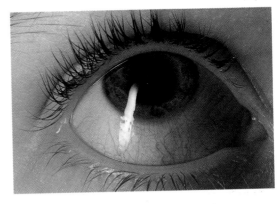

Fig. 6.3 Episcleritis. The deep localized redness and swelling of the episcleral tissue can be seen.

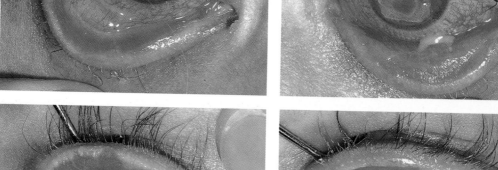

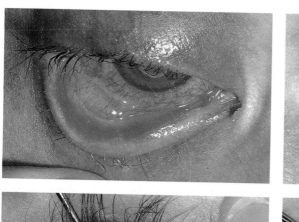

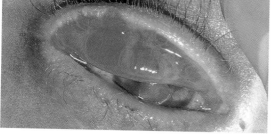

Fig. 6.4 Stevens–Johnson syndrome. Bilateral desquamative conjunctivitis with areas of necrosis. There is a severe keratitis which resulted in chronic scarring, worsened by the later occurrence of a dry eye.

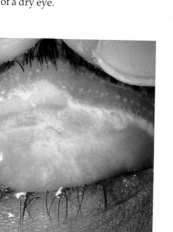

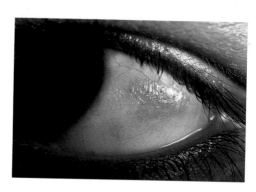

Fig. 6.6 Xerophthalmia. Bitot's spots are flaky elevated patches in the exposed areas of the conjunctiva. As in this case they are often pigmented. (By courtesy of Mr. Michael Eckstein.)

Fig. 6.5 Stevens–Johnson syndrome. Late-stage with subconjunctival scarring, and squamous metaplasia of the lid margins.

Episcleritis
- Moderately deep redness of the conjunctiva and episcleral tissue (Fig. 6.3).
- May be nodular.
- Irritation.
- Treatment is with oral and topical non-steroidal anti-inflammatory agents.
- Steroids may help in resistant cases.

Erythema multiforme (Stevens–Johnson syndrome)
Onset
Follows infections, especially herpes simplex, or drug sensitivity, particularly sulphonamides.
- Widespread skin eruption with 'target' lesions (raised blue/red tender, coin-sized areas).
- Mucous membrane redness swelling, sloughing.
- Conjunctival involvement:
    (a) conjunctivitis;
    (b) mucoid discharge;
    (c) papillary reaction;
    (d) conjunctival infarction (Fig. 6.4);
    (e) membrane formation, conjunctival infarction;
    (f) symblepharon;
    (g) bacterial suprainfection.

Late changes
- Scarring.
- Lacrimal canalicular obstruction.
- Dry eye.
- Keratitis.
- Corneal vascularization and scarring.
- Lid cicatrization and keratinization (Fig. 6.5).

Management
Acute phase
- Admission to hospital.
- Systemic steroids.
- Skin care.
- Intensive topical preservative-free steroids.
- Topical preservative-free antibiotics.
- Cycloplegics.
- Separation of adhesions with a glass rod.

Chronic phase
- Dry eyes may be managed by lubricants (see Chapter 12).
- Topical retinoid treatment for keratinization.
- Epilation, cryotherapy for trichiasis.
- Surgical treatment for entropion.

Aetiology
Probably an acute hypersensitivity reaction.

Avitaminosis A
- One of the most common causes of blindness throughout the world.
- Associated with protein-calorie malnutrition.
- Follows night blindness.
- Dry wrinkled dull conjunctiva (Fig. 6.6).
- Bitot's spots in exposed areas.
- Dry eye.
- Liquefactive acute keratitis occurs with rapid corneal perforation.

Non-infective keratitis
See Chapter 11.

7: Disorders of the Eye as a Whole

Anophthalmos

Clinical anophthalmos is the term used when there is no eye visible on clinical examination. There may be a very small eye that is barely visible and there is a spectrum of conditions from microphthalmos through to anophthalmos.

• Most cases are sporadic, of unknown cause and clusters have been reported (Fig. 7.1).

• It may occur as a part of extreme microphthalmos in families with colobomatous microphthalmos (see Chapter 18) (Figs 7.2 & 7.3).

• Other causes: environmental agents such as X-rays and drugs taken during the pregnancy (LSD), but with these it is unusual to be able to demonstrate a clear causal relationship.

Clinical assessment

The child needs to be examined to see if there is any response to light such as a startle response to a photograph flash gun, and visual evoked potentials (VEPs) may be helpful in being able to determine any residual function. The shape and size of the orbit are examined to assess the need for orbital expansion procedures. If the condition appears to be unilateral, the 'normal' eye must be examined carefully.

The parents and siblings need to have their anterior segments and optic nerves examined, in particular to exclude coloboma.

Management

• The stimulation of orbital growth by orbital implants, increasing sizes of artificial eyes and, in older cases, surgery.

• Parental support, early stimulation of any residual vision, early intervention to encourage general development and early consideration of the best type of education for the child.

Microphthalmos

Microphthalmos is demonstrated when the axial length of the eye is two standard deviations below the normal, i.e. 21 mm in an adult or 19 mm in a 1 year old.

The effect of microphthalmos on vision depends on its extent, and the presence of any associated anomalies. Some microphthalmic eyes may have normal vision, but most severely affected cases have very poor vision; it is important to avoid making inappropriately premature predictions of visual function based solely on the size of the eye.

Isolated microphthalmos

• Idiopathic.
• Inherited:
  (a) autosomal dominant;
  (b) autosomal recessive;
  (c) X-linked recessive.

Microphthalmos with ocular abnormalities

This is associated with the following.

1 Two segment developmental abnormalities, i.e. Peter's, Reiger's, etc.

2 Cataract.

3 Persistent hyperplastic vitreous (PHPV).

4 Retinal disease, i.e. retinopathy of prematurity (ROP), retinal dysplasia, retinal folds, etc.

5 Aniridia.

6 Colobomatous microphthalmos. Coloboma is a frequent association either in isolated microphthalmos or in microphthalmos with systemic disease.

Microphthalmos with systemic disease

1 Temple Al-Gazali syndrome: microphthalmos, dermal aplasia and sclerocornea with Xp22.2-PTER deletion.

2 Chromosomal syndromes. Most of these are asso-

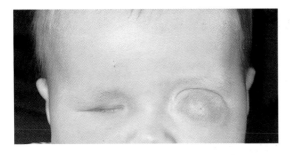

Fig. 7.1 Microphthalmos with cyst (left eye). Clinical anophthalmos (right eye). This baby had presented at birth with a clinically anophthalmic right eye and extreme colobomatous microphthalmos in the left eye. A blue swelling was initially thought to be a vascular anomaly but it transilluminated and was found to be a cyst associated with the microphthalmos.

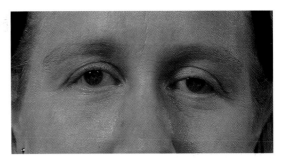

Fig. 7.2 Bilateral non-colobomatous microphthalmos in an adult.

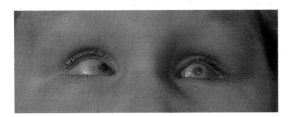

Fig. 7.3 The child of the patient in Fig. 7.2 was born with bilateral marked microphthalmos. Autosomal dominant inheritance is frequent.

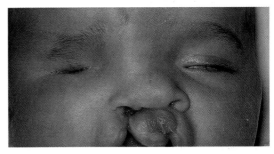

Fig. 7.4 Bilateral microphthalmos, extreme on the right, in a patient with a bilateral cleft palate.

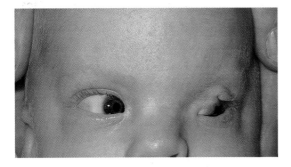

Fig. 7.5 Fraser's syndrome. Partial cryptophthalmos in the left eye. The eye is small and the cornea is partially opaque. The left upper lid is colobomatous and partly fused to the eye. There is often an extended hairline down to the brow. Note the ipsilateral nose deformity.

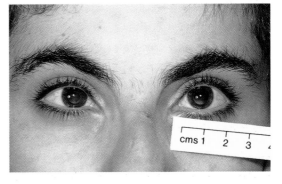

Fig. 7.6 Nanophthalmos showing small eyes with an abnormal fundus reflex due to the high hypermetropia. The anterior chambers are shallow (not visible in this picture) and the eyes are prone to angle closure glaucoma. The optic discs are often crowded and there is prominent foveal yellow pigment with a fold between the fovea and the optic disc.

ciated with colobomas: these syndromes can be found in Chapter 18.

3 Mental retardation.
4 Macrosomia: cleft palate.
5 Facial defects:
  (a) midline brain defect (Fig. 7.4);
  (b) the branchio-oculo-facial syndrome;
  (c) the fronto-facio-nasal dysplasia.
6 Delleman's syndrome: skin tags, punched out skin lesions on ears, mental retardation, hydrocephalus, orbital cysts and others.
7 Ectodermal dysplasia.
8 Fetal infections.
9 Fetal toxins.

Clinical assessment
• Visual assessment.
• Refraction.
• Electrophysiology for visual assessment.
• General clinical assessment for associated malformations.
• Cosmetic contact lens wear.
• Low-vision appliances.

Microphthalmos with orbital cyst

This is a condition which is (usually extreme) colobomatous microphthalmos, and is associated with an orbital cyst which increases in size, usually causing a swelling in the lower lid that is transillu-minant (see Fig. 7.1). The cyst is connected to the eye and its removal carries the risk of damage to the eye.

Cryptophthalmos

1 *Complete cryptophthalmos.* The eyes are covered with a layer of skin with no lashes or lid glands. There is no conjunctival sac.
2 *Incomplete cryptophthalmos.* The lids are colobomatous and may be fused with the cornea. The eye is small. Fraser's syndrome includes cryptophthalmos, syndactyly, nose deformities, extension of the hair line towards the brow and the patients are usually mentally retarded (Fig. 7.5).

Nanophthalmos

Nanophthalmos is a special form of microphthalmos characterized by the eye being small, highly hypermetropic with a very thick sclera. There is a tendency towards angle closure glaucoma and uveal effusion, especially related to intraocular surgery (Fig. 7.6).

Cycloplopia and synophthalmos

These are conditions where the two eyes develop together instead of separately. Vision is usually very poor and there are associated severe brain defects.

8: Disorders of the Eyelids and Brows

Congenital lid abnormalities

1 Cryptophthalmos (see Chapter 7).
2 Ablepharon:
   (a) complete absence of the lids;
   (b) associated with
      (i) Neu Laxova syndrome
      (ii) ablepharon macrosomia syndrome.
3 Coloboma:
   (a) isolated;
   (b) associated with facial clefts, i.e. Goldenhar's syndrome (Fig. 8.1), Treacher–Collins syndrome;
   (c) if large, may require primary repair.
4 Ankyloblepharon:
   (a) fused lids;
   (b) narrow palpebral aperture;
   (c) may be autosomal dominant.
5 Ankyloblepharon filiforme adnatum:
   (a) tag-like fusion of the upper and lower lid, usually centrally;
   (b) otherwise normal palpebral fissure.
6 Euryblepharon:
   (a) large palpebral aperture;
   (b) may be autosomal dominant;
   (c) sometimes associated with Down's syndrome or craniofacial dysostoses.
7 Congenital ectropion:
   (a) associated with
      (i) blepharophimosis
      (ii) Down's syndrome
      (iii) craniofacial syndromes
      (iv) lamellar ichthyosis;
   (b) treated by lubrication, short-term temporary tarsorrhaphy or surgery;
   (c) acute ectropion is known as eversion.
8 Epiblepharon:
   (a) a fold of skin across the upper or lower eyelid, forcing lashes against the cornea;
   (b) common in Orientals (Fig. 8.2);
   (c) improves spontaneously, rarely requires treatment;
   (d) treatment required for associated keratitis—skin elapse excision usually effective.
9 Entropion (Fig. 8.3):
   (a) secondary to microphthalmos;
   (b) secondary to orbicularis spasm;
   (c) Larsen's syndrome
      (i) multiple joint dislocations
      (ii) dysmorphism, cleft palate
      (iii) mental retardation;
   (d) tarsal kink—a horizontal congenital distortion of the tarsus.
Short-term temporary tarsorrhaphy; surgery is occasionally necessary.
10 Epicanthus (Fig. 8.4):
   (a) epicanthic folds are folds of skin extending from the upper or lower lid towards the medial canthus or from the medial canthus, medially;
   (b) common in Orientals;
   (c) marked in the blepharophimosis syndrome.
11 Telecanthus (Fig. 8.5):
   (a) increased width between the medial canthi;
   (b) if required, can be improved by shortening the medial canthal tendons.
12 Blepharophimosis:
   (a) small horizontal palpebral apertures;
   (b) the blepharophimosis syndrome
      (i) ptosis
      (ii) telecanthus
      (iii) blepharophimosis
      (iv) epicanthus inversus — autosomal dominant, 50% sporadic (mostly new mutations), gene locus at 3q22.3–q23, females may be relatively infertile, strabismus frequent.

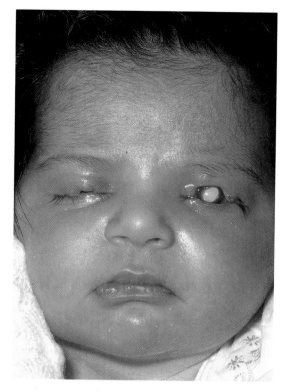

Fig. 8.1 Bilateral lid colobomas in a patient with Goldenhar's syndrome. This child had corneal exposure on the left side.

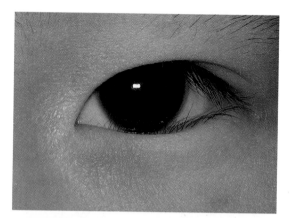

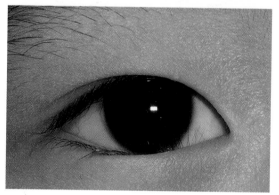

Fig. 8.2 Epiblepharon. In this child the lower lid lashes have turned in from birth. Spontaneous improvement usually occurs.

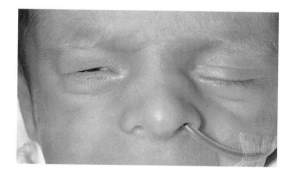

Fig. 8.3 Congenital entropion. This child presented with irritability and an abnormality of the right lids which were slightly swollen. The right upper lid shows entropion with the lashes inturned and abrading the cornea without damage at this stage. It was treated with simple lid suture and it resolved without complication.

Box 8.1 Lid retraction in infancy

1 Physiological.
2 Idiopathic.
3 Pseudo-ipsilateral proptosis or contralateral ptosis.
4 Bilateral in 'setting sun sign' in hydrocephalus.
5 Marcus Gunn jaw winking.
6 Neonatal Graves' disease.
7 Myasthenia.
8 Third nerve palsy with aberrant degeneration.
9 Myopathies.
10 Seventh nerve palsy.
11 Levator fibrosis.
12 Vertical lid-associated nystagmus.

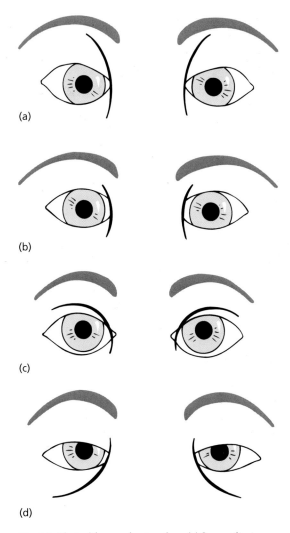

(a)

(b)

(c)

(d)

Fig. 8.4 Clinical forms of epicanthus. (a) Superciliaris, (b) polpebralis, (c) tarsalis, (d) inversus.

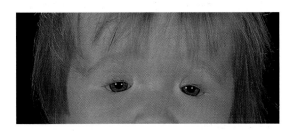

Fig. 8.5 Telecanthus and epicanthus inversus.

Ptosis

Congenital ptosis

1 Dystrophic—simple congenital ptosis (Fig. 8.6):
   (a) most common;
   (b) dystrophic levator muscle;
   (c) lid lag on downgaze;
   (d) variably reduced skin crease;
   (e) often an associated superior rectus weakness;
   (f) found in association with blepharophimosis syndrome (see above) (Fig. 8.7).
2 Non-dystrophic ptosis:
   (a) no lid lag on downgaze;
   (b) good levator function.
3 Congenital neurogenetic ptosis:
   (a) usually third nerve palsy;

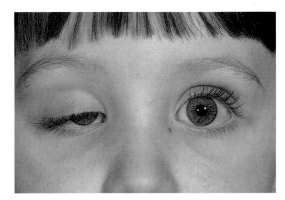

Fig. 8.6 Unilateral simple congenital ptosis.

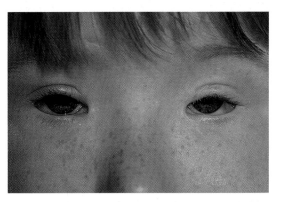

Fig. 8.7 Blepharophimosis syndrome. Bilateral treated ptosis, telecanthus and blepharophimosis.

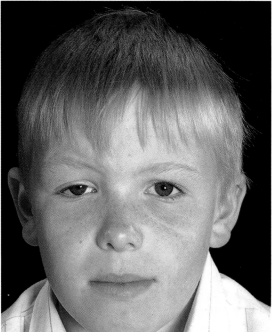

(a)

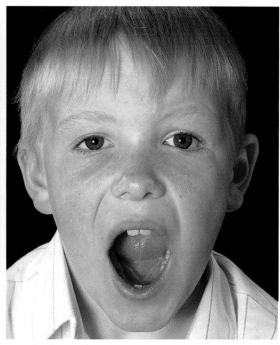

(b)

Fig. 8.8 Marcus Gunn jaw winking phenomenon. (a) Moderate ptosis; (b) with jaw open the right upper lid rises.

   (b) aberrant regeneration—the ptosis may elevate when the patient adducts, depresses or elevates the affected eye;
   (c) cyclic third nerve palsy;
   (d) lid mostly paretic;
   (e) in the 'spastic phase' the eyelid elevates, the pupil becomes small and the eye may adduct;
   (f) periodicity varies as spastic phase usually lasts less than 1 minute.
4 Marcus Gunn jaw winking phenomenon:
   (a) ptosis usually present;
   (b) lid opens when jaw opened or deviated to opposite side, or with swallowing;
   (c) caused by pterygoid synkinesis (Fig. 8.8).

Acquired ptosis
1 Aponeurotic defects:
   (a) blepharochalasis;

   (b) recurrent lid oedema;
   (c) acquired aponeurotic defect;
   (d) lid skin finely wrinkled;
   (e) often bilateral.
2 Neurogenic:
   (a) third nerve palsy;
   (b) Horner's syndrome
      (i) mild ptosis
      (ii) lower lid may also be elevated
      (iii) miosis
      (iv) ipsilateral anhydrosis;
   (c) congenital Horner's syndrome:
      (i) may be due to birth difficulties with the use of forceps;
      (ii) usually idiopathic;
   (d) acquired Horner's syndrome—usually a sign of sympathetic damage often by thoracic surgery, neuroblastoma in infancy or thoracic outlet tumours in childhood.
3 Myogenic ptosis:
   (a) myasthenia gravis
      (i) often asymmetrical

(ii) may be congenital if mother affected, then it is transient

(iii) may be infantile onset

(iv) thymic hypoplasia or thymic tumour present

(v) associated eye muscle abnormality and diplopia

(vi) orbicularis oculi often weak

(vii) diagnosis helped by Tensilon (edrophonium test);

Box 8.2 Tensilon test

The following applies to an adult-sized child. Smaller children must have the dosage reduced appropriately.

1 The test is carried out in a situation where cardiopulmonary rescucitation is readily available.

2 The ptosis or strabismus or eye movements are measured.

3 2 mg of Tensilon (edrophonium hydrochloride) are given intravenously, waiting 5 minutes for abnormal reactions or improvement in the ptosis or eye movement abnormality.

4 After 5 minutes, 8 mg is given intravenously over 1–2 seconds.

5 An improvement in the ptosis, eye position or movement measurements may be taken as a positive response.

6 Side-effect — vasovagal attack — this may be treated or prevented with intramuscular or intravenous atropine.

(b) Progressive external ophthalmoplegia (Fig. 8.9)—may present in later childhood;

(c) Mechanical ptosis — lid tumours, scar tissue, etc.

4 Pseudoptosis:

(a) defective eye elevation—the contralateral eye and lid elevate but the ipsilateral eye and lid are unable to do so;

(b) blepharochalasis occurs when the lid skin becomes lax, as in old age and when there has been an upper lid haemangioma.

Treatment of ptosis

1 A full ocular examination and measurement of the ptosis and lid excursion is mandatory. It is important to note whether the eye movements and position are normal and if Bell's phenomenon is present.

2 Treatment is usually surgical if indicated for cosmetic or functional reasons. Mild ptosis can be treated by a Fasanella–Servat procedure where the upper border of the tarsal plate and the lower part of Muller's muscle is clamped and excised.

3 Moderate congenital ptosis is usually treated by a form of levator shortening procedure. The posterior approach is cosmetically the most acceptable but the anterior approach allows a greater levator resection. Large resections give rise to lid lag on downgaze and there may be some degree of closure defect at night.

4 Severe ptosis is usually treated by a levator suspension material either using autogenous fascia lata or a synthetic material (Fig. 8.10).

5 When there is an associated strabismus it is best to treat this first, especially if there is a vertical element.

6 Myogenic ptosis often produces unsatisfactory results and gives a risk of exposure, especially since Bell's phenomenon is often abnormal.

Lid tumours

Haemangioma

- Common.
- Early onset.
- Rapid initial growth.
- Underlying astigmatism ('plus' axis 90° to the tumour).

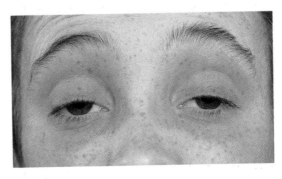

Fig. 8.9 Bilateral ptosis and brow elevation in chronic external ophthalmoplegia.

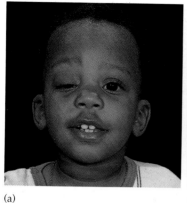
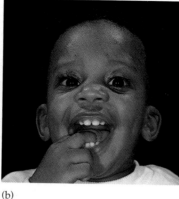

(a)   (b)

Fig. 8.10 (a) Severe unilateral ptosis. There is a marked right ptosis with no skin crease. The child has received occlusion of the left eye since shortly after birth and this has improved the acuity to normal levels. (b) Same child postoperatively. A bilateral levator sling procedure has been carried out: the skin marks of which can be seen on both brows and forehead.

• Spontaneous improvement always occurs with time.
• Surgery usually contraindicated unless very well demarcated.
• May improve with systemic or intralesional depot steroid injection (Fig. 8.11).
• Surgery to improve residual skin lesions after spontaneous involution.
• Tuneable dye laser treatment for superficial elements may be helpful.
• Amblyopia is the biggest cause of visual defect in these cases and occlusion therapy is mandatory in nearly every case together with optical correction where possible.

Box 8.3 Local steroid injections for haemangiomas

1 4 mg of triamcinolone and/or 40 mg depomedrone.
2 Needle inserted deep into the haemangioma.
3 The syringe plunger is withdrawn to ensure that intravascular injection will not occur.
4 Very slow injection into the haemangioma, slowly withdrawing the needle.
5 Care must be taken to watch for superficial tracking of the depot preparation, which will leave white lines on the skin for many months.
6 Injection may be repeated after 3–6 weeks.
7 If no improvement, only two rounds of injections are given.
8 If improvement occurs, a further injection is given when the shrinkage seems to have stopped.

Other tumours, granulomas, etc.
• Naevi.
• Internal and external angle dermoid cysts.
• Molluscum contagiosum: lid margin lesions may require curettage and diathermy because they cause a conjunctivitis (Fig. 8.12).
• Juvenile xanthogranuloma.
• Calcifying epithelioma of Malherbe, which is small, hard and benign.

Inflammatory lid disease

• Meibomianitis.
• Meibomian cyst. Most meibomian cysts resolve spontaneously; they may be helped by massage and lid toilet with very dilute solutions of baby shampoo twice a day or treatment with topical antibiotic ointment.
• Incision and curettage can be carried out for large refractory cases.
• Acute blepharitis (Fig. 8.13).
• *Staphylococcus aureus* or other bacterial infection.
• Ulcerations around lash margins, etc., respond well to local antibiotic and lid toilet.

Chronic blepharitis
• Irritable lids.
• Itching.
• Lid swelling.
• Associated red eyes.
• Respond to lid toilet and short courses of antibiotic lid ointment.

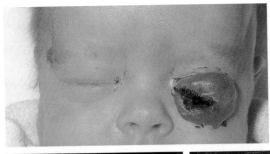

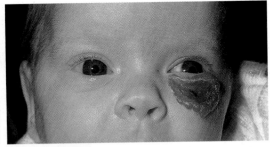

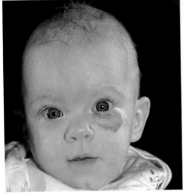

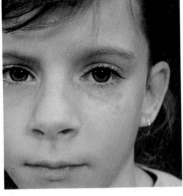

Fig. 8.11 Haemangioma of the lower lid. This presented as a rapidly increasing mass in the left lower lid which occluded the eye by the age of 6 weeks. It was treated with three separate injections of depot steroid and resolved leaving minimal skin changes.

- Chronic or acute blepharitis.
- Post-irradiation.

Trichiasis
- Backward turning lashes with normal positioned margins:
    (a) lid fibrosis;
    (b) trachoma;

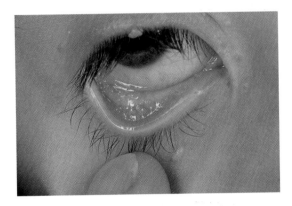

Fig. 8.12 Molluscum contagiosum showing multiple lesions and a follicular conjunctivitis.

Abnormalities of lashes

Absence of lashes
- Ichthyosis.
- Alopecia.
- Trichotillomania (psychogenic lash or brow plucking).

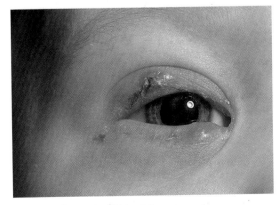

Fig. 8.13 Acute blepharitis with lid ulceration and stye formation.

(c) Stevens–Johnson syndrome;
(d) burns, etc.
- Treatment involves electrolysis or cryotherapy as in distichiasis.

Distichiasis
- Second row of lashes growing from the meibomian glands.
- Isolated.
- Falls–Kertesz syndrome: lymphoedema of the legs plus distichiasis.
- Other rare syndromes.
- Treatment involves repeated epilation or electrolysis, or lid splitting with cryotherapy to the posterior lamella.

Eyebrows

Synophrys
- Eyebrows which join medially.

- Cornelia de Lang syndrome.
- Waardenburg syndrome.
- Some mucopolysaccharidoses.
- Other rare syndromes.

Sparse or absent eyebrows
- Ablepharon macrostomia syndrome.
- Alopecia.
- Trichotillomania.
- Ectodermal dysplasia.
- Ichthiosis.
- Trichomegaly syndrome.
- Progeria.
- Hallermann–Streiff–François syndrome.

9: Orbital Disease

Orbital disease in children

Clinical disorders of the orbit in childhood may result from developmental anomalies or may be acquired from orbital disease. Children with acquired orbital diseases most commonly present with signs and symptoms of a mass within the orbit. These signs may include:
- reduced vision;
- restriction of ocular movement;
- pain and inflammation;
- proptosis.

In children structural abnormalities (including cysts) and neoplasia account for the great majority of orbital disease. In contrast, in adults over 50% are due to inflammatory causes and less than 20% are due to structural abnormalities.

When assessing a child with orbital disease, a careful history and examination will usually limit the differential diagnosis considerably. The age of onset, laterality and a temporal onset of the orbital problem are important historical factors.

The ophthalmological examination of the child should include:
- visual acuity assessment;
- ocular motor assessment;
- measurement of proptosis;
- slit lamp examination;
- pupillary examination (especially for afferent pupillary assessment);
- cycloplegic refraction;
- funduscopic examination;
- systemic examination (especially important in suspected cases of neurofibromatosis, juvenile xanthogranuloma and Langerhan's cell histiocytosis).

Most children with orbital pathology will require some form of neuroradiological investigation. These may include:

- plain X-rays;
- sinus X-rays;
- computerized tomography (CT) scanning;
- magnetic resonance imaging (MRI).

Inflammatory diseases

The principle causes of inflammation of the orbit in children may be divided into non-specific orbital inflammatory syndromes (NSOIS) (previously referred to as orbital pseudotumour) and specific causes (such as sarcoidosis and Wegener's granulomatosis). These become increasingly more common in the second decade of life when orbital diseases in childhood begin to resemble those found in adults.

NSOIS

These acute or subacute inflammatory disorders of the orbit of unknown cause may take on several forms depending upon the site of inflammation.

1 *Anterior idiopathic orbital inflammation.* This is the most common type of NSOIS occurring in childhood. The pathology is confined to the anterior orbit and adjacent globe. The patient may present with:
   (a) pain;
   (b) proptosis;
   (c) lid swelling;
   (d) conjunctival infection;
   (e) decreased vision;
   (f) anterior and posterior uveitis (Fig. 9.1).

2 *Diffuse idiopathic orbital inflammation.* This is similar to the anterior form although it is often more severe and is characterized by:
   (a) more severe restriction of eye movement;
   (b) more pronounced visual acuity loss due to retinal detachment or optic atrophy;
   (c) inflammatory changes that are diffuse throughout the orbit (Fig. 9.2).

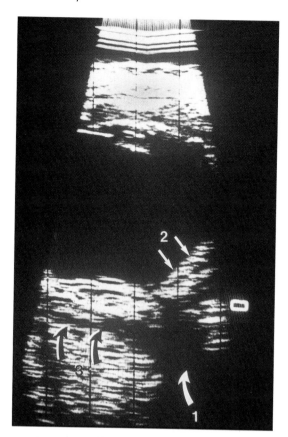

Fig. 9.1 Ultrascan of a patient with anterior NSOIS showing the so-called T sign. There is doubling of the optic nerve shadow, shallow retinal detachment and accentuation of Tenon's space. Patient of Dr Jack Rootman.

3 *Idiopathic orbital myositis.* This inflammatory disorder is characterized by:

(a) pain and limitation of eye movement (usually paresis of the involved muscle);

(b) diplopia;

(c) ptosis;

(d) lid oedema;

(e) conjunctival chemosis;

(f) proptosis may also occur (Fig. 9.3).

Neuroimaging studies reveal enlargement of the muscle and tendon in contradistinction to thyroid orbitopathy where the tendon is usually spared.

4 *Idiopathic lacrimal inflammation.* This relatively well-localized form of inflammation presents with:

(a) pain, tenderness and swelling over the upper lid;

(b) ptosis and an 'S'-shaped deformity of the lid;

(c) globe displacement downward and medially;

(d) superiotemporal conjunctival chemosis;

(e) no uveitis.

Neuroimaging studies reveal the inflammation to be centred on the lacrimal gland but often involving the adjacent side of the globe.

Almost all forms of non-specific orbital inflammation respond to steroids although the anterior and diffuse forms may require much more prolonged therapy than the myositis or idiopathic lacrimal form.

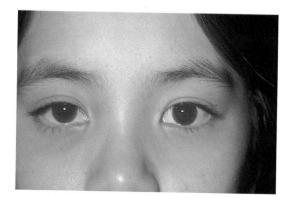

Fig. 9.2 A patient with diffuse NSOIS who presented with a retrobulbar ache, associated with ptosis and pain on eye movement.

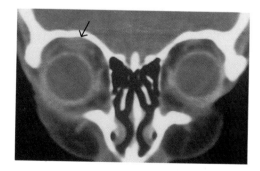

Fig. 9.3 Left superior rectus myositis in a 16-year-old boy. Ptosis and painful limitation of upgaze with diplopia were the presenting signs. This was due to left superior rectus myositis seen as a thickened muscle complex on the CT scan. Patient of Dr Jack Rootman.

Specific causes of orbital inflammation

1 *Wegener's granulomatosis.* This is a necrotizing granulomatous vasculitis that has a predilection for the airway and kidneys. It is rare in children.

2 *Sarcoidosis.* This granulomatous inflammatory disease of unknown cause may cause optic nerve infiltration, uveitis, extraocular muscle infiltration or lacrimal gland enlargement. It has been reported infrequently in teenagers.

3 *Thyroid orbitopathy.* Although this may be a common cause of proptosis in older children, thyroid orbitopathy in children appears to be milder than in adults. Thus, optic neuropathy, sight-threatening corneal problems and severe extraocular muscle involvement are characteristically less common.

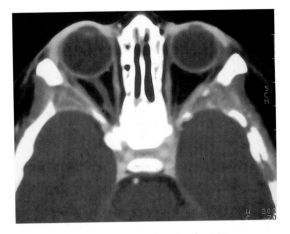

Fig. 9.4 A case of Langerhan's cell histiocytosis with extensive orbital involvement with bony erosion seen on CT scan.

Histiocytic, haematopoietic and lymphoproliferative disorders

Three histiocyte disorders may involve the eye and orbits.

1 *Langerhan's cell histiocytosis (histiocytosis X).* This is an uncommon disorder characterized by focal proliferation of abnormal histiocytes within different tissues. Tissues that may be affected include:

(a) skin;
(b) bone;
(c) spleen;
(d) liver;
(e) lymph nodes;
(f) lung.

Ophthalmic involvement is common and may affect a number of different structures including:

(a) uvea—most frequently seen in infants;
(b) optic nerves, chiasm or tract;
(c) third, fourth, fifth or sixth cranial nerves;
(d) orbit — usually affects parietal and frontal bone, producing a lytic lesion (Fig. 9.4).

This disorder, when function is threatened, may be treated with systemic local depomedrone, steroids or radiotherapy depending upon the tissues involved. Children with single system disease (e.g. involving bone only) have a good prognosis. In contrast, the prognosis is poor in multisystem or visceral disease. Children under the age of 2 years (who are most likely to have multisystem disease) have a mortality rate of 50–60%; death is rare in older children.

2 *Non-Langerhan's cell histiocytosis.* Juvenile xanthogranuloma is a disorder of unknown aetiology in which there is an abnormal proliferation of non-Langerhan's histiocytes. Characteristically it involves the skin, with less than 5% of patients demonstrating ocular involvement. It may involve the iris, ciliary body or posterior choroid. Typically, the iris lesion is yellow or creamy white and is associated with the risk of spontaneous hyphaema and glaucoma (Fig. 9.5). Systemic steroids may be effective. Orbital and epibulbar involvement is uncommon.

3 *Sinus histiocytosis.* Sinus histiocytosis is a disease of unknown aetiology, primarily affecting children and young adults. It is characterised by massive, painless cervical lymphadenopathy with extranodule involvement being seen in the orbit, upper respiratory tract, salivary gland, skin, testes and bone.

The condition affects the soft tissues of the orbit without bony involvement. Progressive proptosis without optic nerve compromise may occur.

Treatment with high-dose steroids, systemic chemotherapy and radiotherapy have all been reported.

4 *Leukaemia*: see Chapter 23.

5 *Lymphoma*: see Chapter 23.

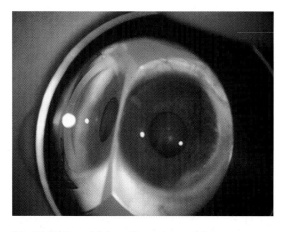

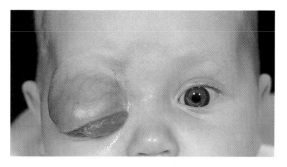

Fig. 9.6 Capillary haemangioma of the anterior orbit and lid. They often increase in size on straining.

Fig. 9.5 Patient with juvenile xanthogranuloma. Gonioscopy view showing the angle filled with yellowish xanthogranuloma material. It can also be seen in the bottom right of the picture.

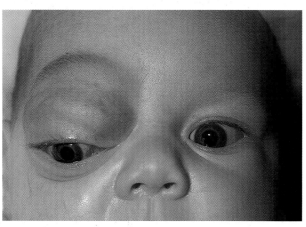

(a)

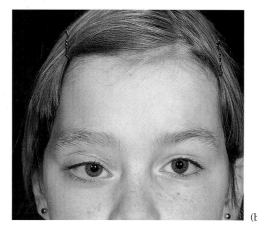

(b)

Fig. 9.7 (a) Orbital capillary haemangioma in a child aged 2 months. (b) Same patient aged 9 years after some spontaneous resolution and surgery. Surgery is usually not necessary and best avoided in most circumstances.

Vascular disease

Tumours

A number of different vascular tumours may involve the orbit. These include the following.

Capillary haemangioma

Capillary haemangioma is the most common orbital tumour in childhood. It occurs more frequently in girls than boys. Characteristically, spontaneous regression occurs. The clinical features of capillary haemangiomas are:

- most commonly situated in the upper lid or orbit (Fig. 9.6);
- rapid growth during the first few months of life followed by a slower period of regression;
- proptosis;
- amblyopia, usually secondary to anisometropia but occasionally to strabismus or form deprivation (as a result of severe ptosis).

Since spontaneous regression is the rule, treatment is indicated only if amblyopia is suspected (Fig. 9.7).

Treatment
See Chapter 8.

Haemangiopericytoma
This rare tumour, derived from pericytes, is usually seen in adults. It is locally invasive and may give rise to distant metastases. Its usual clinical presentation is with gradual increasing proptosis.

Lymphohaemangioma
These vascular lesions commonly arise in childhood and may be difficult to distinguish from haemangioma. In contrast to capillary haemangioma, however, neither marked growth nor spontaneous regression usually occur. The lesions may be superficial, involving the preseptal lid tissue or deep within the orbit presenting as proptosis. Conservative management is indicated unless visual compromise is documented.

Congenital orbital varices
Without orbital contrast studies, orbital varices may be difficult to distinguish from lymphangiomas. Varices typically give rise to recurrent haemorrhage with sudden increased proptosis. Conservative management is usually indicated unless massive proptosis persists (Fig. 9.8).

Sturge–Weber syndrome
See Chapter 24.

Klippel–Trenaunay–Weber syndrome
See Chapter 24.

Neurofibromatosis
See Chapter 24.

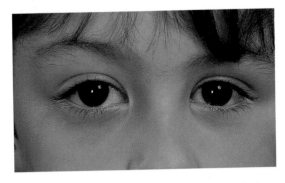

Fig. 9.8 Patient with orbital varices. A subconjunctival varix can just be seen in the right lateral fornix.

Neurogenic tumours

Optic nerve tumours
Gliomas (astrocytomas) may affect the anterior visual pathways either in the orbit or intracranial compartment (Fig. 9.9).

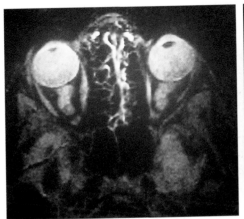

(a)

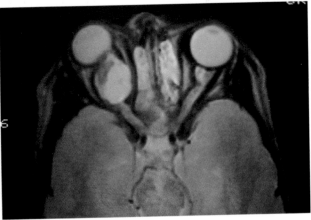

(b)

Fig. 9.9 (a) Bilateral optic nerve glioma in a patient with NF1 who had been followed with no change in vision or neuroimaging for many years. (b) Optic nerve glioma with cystic area anteriorly.

Optic nerve glioma (orbital)

The vast majority of these present in childhood with:

- axial proptosis;
- visual loss secondary to optic atrophy;
- strabismus with or without limitation of ocular movement;
- disc swelling;
- optociliary shunt vessels.

Characteristic radiographic features are:

- kinking of the optic nerve in the immediate retrobulbar zone;
- enlargement of the optic canal when involved.

Optic nerve gliomas are low-grade pilocytic astrocytomas. Treatment remains controversial. Many cases remain stable over long periods of time with no change in visual function (Table 9.1).

Chiasmal gliomas

These are more common than orbital gliomas. Clinical presentation usually consists of:

- bilateral visual loss;
- nystagmus (may mimic spasmus nutans);
- strabismus;
- optic atrophy;
- papilloedema;
- growth failure;
- proptosis is unusual unless optic nerves are also involved (Fig. 9.10).

Treatment, again, remains controversial as many of these patients also appear to be stable over long periods of time. No controversy exists about the need for endocrine assessment and replacement and treatment of hydrocephalus when present. Radiation therapy and chemotherapy have both been advocated in the patient with progressive visual loss.

Meningiomas

Meningiomas are very rare in childhood but may be seen in teenagers.

Table 9.1 Characteristics of optic nerve (ON) glioma with and without neurofibromatosis 1 (NF1). (Courtesy of Mr Christopher Lyons.)

	NF1	No NF1
Associated features	Café au lait spots Lisch nodules Other tumours (see text)	None
Presentation	Asymptomatic Routine examination finding Visual loss	Visual loss Strabismus Proptosis
Tumour distribution	Multifocal, diffuse, bilateral	Discrete, unilateral
Progression	Stable slow progression Fluctuating vision	Stable slow progression Occasionally rapid
Histology	Arachnoid gliomatosis Perineural gliomatosis Mucinous accumulation	Obliteration of perineural space by expanding ON
Radiographic findings	Fusiform ON enlargement High signal intensity in perineural arachnoid gliomatosis on T2-weighted MRI Kinking of intra-orbital nerve	Fusiform ON enlargement Loss of perineural space
Visual prognosis	Good	Poor
Life expectancy	Reduced mostly from other tumours	Normal

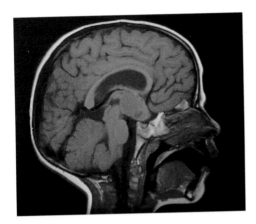

Fig. 9.10 Chiasmal and hypothalamic glioma with thickened intracranial optic nerves.

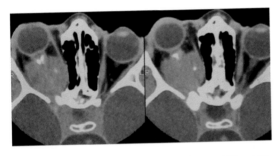

Fig. 9.11 Optic nerve meningioma in a 5-year-old boy. CT scan showing calcification around the optic nerve and orbital expansion.

Optic nerve sheath meningioma

These present with:
• visual loss;
• mild or no proptosis;
• strabismus and diplopia;
• optic atrophy;
• optociliary shunt vessels—common (Fig. 9.11).

Visual loss may be early and profound when these tumours are intracanalicular. Treatment is rarely indicated although surgical excision and radiation therapy are occasionally utilized. This is often associated with NF2.

Extraoptic meningioma

When these involve the sphenoid wing, suprasellar area or olfactory groove, compression of the anterior visual pathway with visual loss may occur. These are uncommon in children.

Rhabdomyosarcomas

Primary orbital malignant tumours are extremely rare in children; rhabdomyosarcoma is the most common. Most appear after the age of 4 years and before the age of 10 years but have been reported in infancy. Familial cases have been reported and related to mutations of *p53* gene, situated on the short arm of chromosome 17.

Clinical features include:
• proptosis which may be sudden and progressive, over a few days;
• eyelid erythema and oedema;
• ophthalmoplegia;
• ptosis;
• palpable lid mass.

Rhabdomyosarcomas spread virtually only by local invasion, but involvement of the anterior or middle cranial fossa, pterygopalatine fossa or nasal cavity may occur (Fig. 9.12).

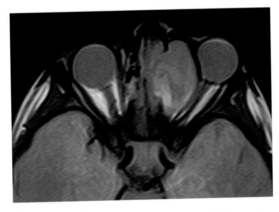

Fig. 9.12 This 20-month-old girl had a 3-week history of left proptosis, nasal discharge and nose bleeds. There is a 7-mm proptosis of the left eye with 5 mm of lateral globe displacement. On MRI, an ethmoidal mass had eroded through the medial orbital wall and displaced the orbital contents anterior and laterally. The mass had also obstructed the nasal cavity. Intranasal biopsy demonstrated alveolar rhabdomyosarcoma. Patient of Mr Christopher Lyons

CT typically shows a non-enhancing, poorly defined mass of homogeneous density. Biopsy is indicated to establish the diagnosis. Based on histopathology, rhabdomyosarcomas have been divided into three groups:

1 anaplastic;
2 monomorphous;
3 mixed.

Long-term survival rates have increased greatly by early detection and improved treatment modalities. Treatment now usually consists of biopsy, or incomplete excision accompanied by chemotherapy or radiation therapy. Because of significant ocular and orbital complications associated with early orbital and ocular irradiation, increasing emphasis is being placed on long-term chemotherapy.

Other mesenchymal abnormalities
Dysplasias

Fibrous dysplasia of the orbit is a rare disorder of unknown aetiology in which replacement of normal bone by cellular fibrous stroma occurs. Presentation is usually in childhood and the clinical features depend upon which orbital wall is primarily involved.

1 Orbital roof:
   (a) proptosis;
   (b) downward displacement of the globe and orbit.
2 Maxilla:
   (a) displacement of the eye upward;
   (b) persistent epiphora.
3 Sphenoid: optic atrophy, if optic canal involved.
4 Sella turcica: chiasmal compression with optic atrophy.

Fibrous dysplasia is seen on radiographic examination as an expansion of normal bone with sclerotic or cystic areas (Fig. 9.13). Treatment is aimed at preventing progressive visual loss due to optic atrophy, and surgical resection of the involved bone is usually indicated.

Bone tumours

• *Reparative granuloma*:
   (a) part of a spectrum of reactive giant cell lesions including aneurysmal bone cyst;

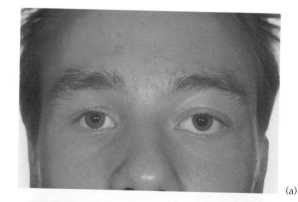
(a)

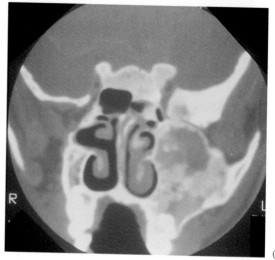
(b)

Fig. 9.13 (a) This 16 year old presented with a history of progressive facial distortion and decreasing visual acuity to 6/18. Compressive optic neuropathy was diagnosed secondary to fibrous dysplasia. (b) The CT scan shows cystic fibrous dysplasia involving the orbital apex, which was decompressed by surgically removing the maxillary component. Patient of Dr Jack Rootman.

   (b) when it involves the sphenoid bones it may lead to proptosis;
   (c) reparative granulomas are treated by surgical resection.
• *Aneurysmal bone cyst*:
   (a) uncommon lesion with infrequent involvement of the orbit;
   (b) most cases involve the orbital roof;
   (c) local surgical resection indicated.

Other mesenchymal tumours

- *Osteoblastoma*:
  (a) benign tumour rarely involving the orbit;
  (b) well-circumscribed lesions;
  (c) surgical treatment indicated.
- *Post-irradiation osteosarcoma of the orbit*:
  (a) occurs in survivors of the genetic form of retinoblastoma;
  (b) extremely poor prognosis.
- *Infantile cortical hyperostosis (Caffey's disease)*:
  (a) uncommon;
  (b) occurs in infancy;
  (c) sudden onset with fever;
  (d) soft tissue swelling over involved bone;
  (e) usually self-limited.
- *Osteopetrosis*:
  (a) rare disorder of bone due to defective resorption;
  (b) may involve the orbits in the autosomal recessive form;
  (c) compressive optic atrophy may occur;
  (d) associated retinal degeneration has been reported (Fig. 9.14).

Metastatic, secondary and lacrimal gland tumours

Neuroblastoma is by far the most common childhood orbital metastatic disease. Other tumours that may be metastatic to the orbit include:

- Ewing's sarcoma;
- Wilm's tumour;
- testicular embryonal sarcoma;
- ovarian sarcoma;
- renal embryonal sarcoma.

Neuroblastoma

Neuroblastoma is the most common solid tumour of childhood with frequent orbital metastases. It is derived from embryonic neural crest tissue. The adrenals are usually the primary site of involvement. The tumour may arise from the cervical sympathetic chain, mediastinum or pelvis. Neuroblastoma is more common in patients with neurofibromatosis type 1.

Ophthalmic features include:

- Horner's syndrome — in mediastinal or cervical sympathetic chain lesions;
- tonic pupils—as a paraneoplastic effect;
- opsoclonus;
- orbital metastases — commonly bilateral with sudden ecchymotic proptosis (Fig. 9.15).

Treatment is usually by surgical resection of any abdominal mass present, usually combined with radiotherapy and chemotherapy. Orbital involvement is usually treated with irradiation or chemotherapy.

Ewing's sarcoma

Ewing's sarcoma is a highly malignant tumour of primitive mesenchyme. It usually arises in the axial skeletal; orbital involvement may be primary or due

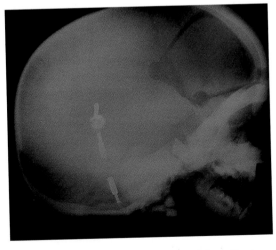

Fig. 9.14 Osteopetrosis. This infant had a bilateral compressive optic neuropathy which failed to respond to optic nerve decompression. He also had a shunt in situ.

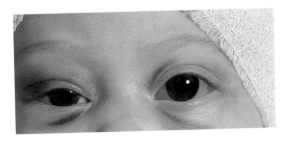

Fig. 9.15 Periorbital ecchymoses in a patient with orbital neuroblastoma.

to spread from contiguous structures. When the orbit is involved, the usual presentation is rapid progressive proptosis with orbital haemorrhage.

On CT scan a moth-eaten appearance of the involved bone is seen.

Treatment of the primary tumour is by irradiation therapy with or without chemotherapy.

Secondary spread

Orbital spread in retinoblastoma has been reduced significantly by early diagnosis and new modalities of treatment (see Chapter 17).

Lacrimal gland tumours

The most common cause of lacrimal gland fossa mass in childhood is dermoid cyst. Both primary epithelial tumours, as well as adenoid cystic carcinoma of the lacrimal gland are uncommon in childhood. These tumours have a tendency to develop rapidly and be associated with pain and paraesthesia due to perineural invasion. Adenoid cystic carcinoma is especially invasive and carries a poor prognosis (Fig. 9.16).

Cystic lesions

Cystic lesions of the orbit in childhood include a number of developmental lesions. In some parts of

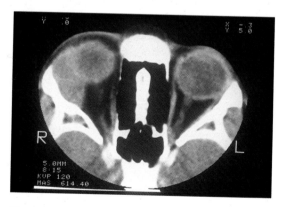

Fig. 9.16 This 10-year-old boy presented with a 1-year history of gradual right orbital enlargement and upper lid swelling. There was no pain or sensory loss. CT scanning showed a lacrimal gland mass excavating the frontal bone without erosion. This was found to be an adenoid cystic carcinoma of the lacrimal gland. The patient is alive and well 10 years later. Patient of Dr Jack Rootman.

the world parasitic cysts such as *Echinococcus* are common.

Lacrimal ductal cyst

These usually occur in adults although they have been reported in teenagers. They involve the palpebral lobe of the lacrimal gland and frequently become apparent following trauma or inflammation of the orbit.

Dermoid cyst

These developmental choristomas that arise from ectodermal arrests are common in childhood. They may be superficial or deep although most are superficial in children.

Superficial dermoids. These present as a rounded mass, typically at the superior temporal margin of the orbit (Fig. 9.17). They are painless, non-tender, firm, non-fluctuant and often immobile.

CT scan findings are characteristic: a round discreet mass associated with thinning and smooth expansion of the underlying bone.

Treatment is by excision.

Deep dermoid. These usually present later in life with gradual involvement and slowly progressive proptosis or globe displacement. Visual loss, strabismus and pain may occur.

CT findings are similar to those of superficial dermoid.

Orbital encephalocoele

These are rare lesions but important since they may be mistaken for a lacrimal sac mucocoele. They arise from an embryological defect in which neuroectoderm fails to separate from surface ectoderm. Cystic herniation of dura and/or brain material into the orbit results. Optic disc anomalies may be associated with them. Anterior orbital encephalocoeles most commonly herniate through the region of the ethmoid but may also occur in the regions of frontal, lacrimal and maxillary bone.

Posterior orbital encephalocoeles herniate via the optic foramen, orbital fissures or a posterior orbital bony defect. They present with slowly progressive proptosis which may be pulsatile.

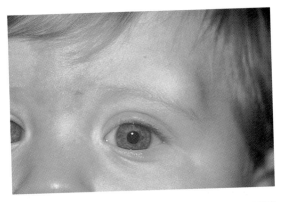

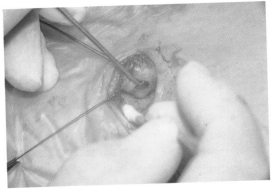

Fig. 9.17 A typical superficial dermoid cyst on the brow of an 18-month-old boy. No intraorbital extension was noted pre-operatively, although a small tail was seen to insert into the bone at the time of surgery. Patient of Mr Christopher Lyons.

Sinus mucocoele

A mucocoele is a cystic swelling of a perinasal sinus which results from obstruction of its osteum. A normal mucous secretion of the respiratory epithelium lining accumulates within the sinus leading to gradual expansion and erosion of its bony walls. Erosion into the orbit or intracranial space may occur.

These are uncommon in childhood since they occur most commonly in the frontal sinus (which does not start to appear in children until the age of 2 years).

Microphthalmos with cyst (Fig. 9.18)

Eyes with severe colobomas and marked microphthalmos may present with an orbital cyst that results from proliferation of neuroectoderm at the lips of

the persistent fetal fissure defect. These are typically seen as a bluish cystic transilluminating lesion in the lower fornix, displacing a microphthalmic or rudimentary eye (see Chapter 7).

Congenital cystic eyeball (anophthalmos with cyst)

Congenital cystic eyeball is distinguished from microphthalmos with cyst by its complete absence of any rudimentary globe.

It presents at birth with large cystic swelling within the affected orbit.

Orbital teratoma

Teratomas are tumours that arise from pluripotential embryonic stem cells and consist of elements derived from one or more germ cell layers.

The usual presentation of a primary orbital teratoma is with unilateral massive proptosis in a newborn child. A normal globe is displaced by a large cystic mass which is often fluctuant and transilluminates. Continuing rapid growth occurs after birth (Fig. 9.19). Exposure keratopathy, ulceration and even perforation of the cornea may occur.

Surgical excision is the preferred treatment.

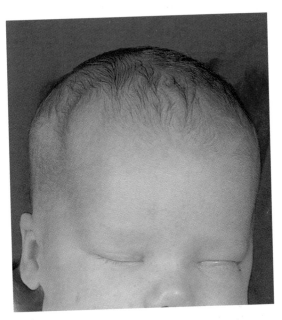

Fig. 9.18 Bilateral microphthalmos with a cyst in the lower lid of the left orbit.

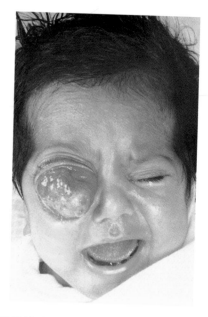

Fig. 9.19 Orbital teratoma.

Craniofacial abnormalities

Craniofacial abnormalities are important to the ophthalmologist because of the frequent associated ocular abnormalities.

Craniosynostosis syndromes

These are syndromes in which an abnormally shaped skull results from premature closure of the suture. They include the following.

1 *Oxycephaly.* This condition is characterised by a high, narrow, pointed or dome-shaped skull. The forehead is high and the superciliary ridges are poorly developed. There is superior prognathism and the palatal arch is high and narrow. The deformity results from premature synostosis of all skull sutures, particularly the coronal sutures. Intracranial hypertension is common.

The ocular features include:
(a) visual failure—with optic atrophy;
(b) proptosis;
(c) strabismus;
(d) amblyopia;
(e) nystagmus (Fig. 9.20).

2 *Crouzon's syndrome.* This autosomal dominant syndrome with complete penetrance but variable expressivity consists of premature craniosynostosis, midfacial hypoplasia and exophthalmos. The gene defect has been mapped to chromosome 10.

The facial appearance is characteristic with orbital shallowing, resulting in proptosis. The nose is

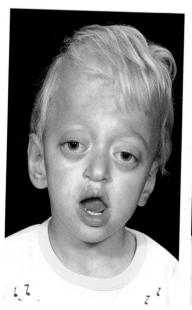
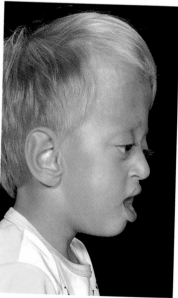

Fig. 9.20 Oxycephaly showing the high narrow skull with increased height of the skull, shallow orbits, superior prognathism and poorly developed superciliary ridges.

hooked and a prominent lower jaw is common. Intracranial hypertension may occur (Fig. 9.21).

Ophthalmic features include:

(a) proptosis—spontaneous subluxation of the globe may occur;

(b) V-pattern exotropia and other forms of strabismus;

(c) optic atrophy or papilloedema;

(d) iris coloboma;

(e) aniridia;

(f) corectopia;

(g) micro- or megalocornea;

(h) cataract;

(i) ectopia lentis;

(j) blue sclera;

(k) glaucoma.

3 *Apert's syndrome.* This syndrome is characterised by craniosynostosis and symmetrical syndactyly of fingers and toes involving the second to fourth and fifth digits. It is inherited as an autosomal dominant disorder with a high spontaneous mutation rate.

Its systemic manifestations include:

(a) high arch palate;

(b) cleft palate;

(c) tracheo-oesophageal fistula;

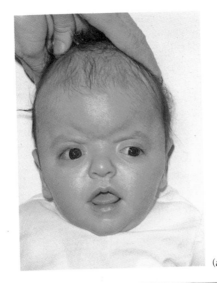

(a)

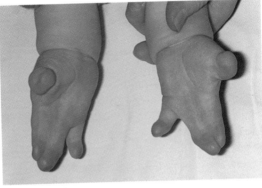

(b)

Fig. 9.22 (a) Apert's syndrome showing the shallow orbits, strabismus and open mouth with maxillary hypoplasia. (b) The syndactyly usually affects the second to fifth digits of hands and feet.

(d) congenital heart disease;

(e) hydrocephalus;

(f) mental retardation (Fig. 9.22).

A typical facial appearance is similar to Crouzon's with a marked deficient supraorbital ridge, midfacial hypoplasia and a prominent lower jaw; dental and ear anomalies including deafness may occur.

The ophthalmic findings may include:

(a) proptosis—usually less marked than Crouzon's;

(b) hypertelorism;

(c) antimongoloid slant of the palpebral fissure;

(d) V-pattern exotropia;

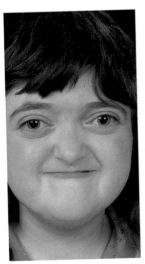 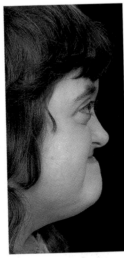

Fig. 9.21 Crouzon's syndrome. This girl has the features of inferior prognathism, maxillary hypoplasia and a prominent forehead. Her nose is quite straight—it is often more 'hooked' in this condition.

(e) optic atrophy or papilloedema;

(f) keratoconus;

(g) ectopia lentis;

(h) congenital glaucoma.

4 *Pfeiffer's syndrome.* This syndrome consists of acrocephaly, mild syndactyly and characteristic broad thumbs and great toes with varus deformities. It is inherited as an autosomal dominant disorder with complete penetrance, but variable expressivity.

Facial and ophthalmic features are similar to Apert's but mental retardation is less common.

5 *Cloverleaf skull.* This appears to be a sporadic disorder. The skull is flat with a trilobed appearance as a result of synostosis of the coronal and lamboidal sutures. The orbits are extremely shallow (Fig. 9.23), proptosis is severe and globe subluxation is a common problem. Hydrocephalus and airway problems are common. Life-expectancy is limited.

6 *Saethre–Chotzen syndrome.* This syndrome consists of a variable skull and facial asymmetry with short fingers, cutaneous syndactyly and low-set frontal hairline. There is very little midfacial hypoplasia and the eyes are not proptopic.

7 *Carpenter's syndrome.* This syndrome consists of craniosynostosis, polysyndactyly of the feet and syndactyly of the hands with shortening of the fingers. The craniosynostosis is severe. Mental retardation is usual. Ocular findings include hypertelorism, epicanthic folds and telecanthus.

Clefting syndromes

These syndromes result from defective apposition or failure of fusion of neighbouring structures during embryonic development. They include the following.

1 *Treacher–Collins syndrome.* This is an autosomal dominant syndrome with complete penetrance but variable expressivity. The gene responsible has been mapped to the long arm of chromosome 5 (5q32–q33.3).

The facial characteristics of this syndrome include:

(a) malar hypoplasia;

(b) hypoplastic zygomas;

(c) absence of nasofrontal angle;

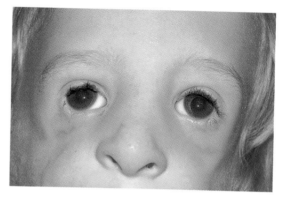

Fig. 9.24 Treacher–Collins syndrome. These patients may have marked malar hypoplasia, an antimongoloid slant to the palpebral fissures and lower lid colobomata. Ear malformations occur and middle and inner ear anomalies may impair hearing.

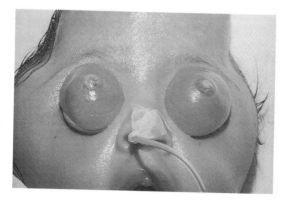

Fig. 9.23 Cloverleaf skull with trilobed flattened skull appearance, subluxed globes, exposure keratitis and chemotic conjunctiva.

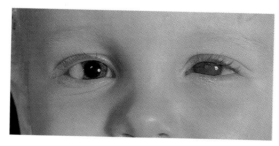

Fig. 9.25 Goldenhar's syndrome showing limbal dermoid on the right and a keratitis due to an anaesthetic cornea on the left.

(d) hypoplasia of the lower jaw;

(e) abnormal dentition;

(f) choanal atresia;

(g) mandibular retrusion (Fig. 9.24).

Malformations of the external ear are common and deafness may occur.

Ophthalmic features include:

(a) palpebral fissures with antimongoloid slant;

(b) colobomas of the lateral third of the lower lid;

(c) canthal dystopia;

(d) nasolacrimal obstruction;

(e) limbal or orbital dermoids.

2 *Goldenhar's syndrome.* This syndrome consists of epibulbar dermoids, pre-auricular appendages and mandibular hypoplasia. Severe hydrocephalus and mental retardation may occur. Vertebral, cardiac, renal and pulmonary anomalies are also common.

Ocular findings include (Fig. 9.25):

(a) ptosis;

(b) nasolacrimal duct obstruction;

(c) coloboma of the mid third of the upper lid;

(d) dermoid or dermolipoma — usually the inferior temporal limbus;

(e) strabismus—including Duane's syndrome.

Management of craniofacial syndromes

These patients have complex cranial, facial, systemic and ophthalmic problems. They need to be managed by a team of paediatricians, neurosurgeons, plastic surgeons, geneticists and ophthalmologists.

Orbital cellulitis

See Chapter 5.

10: Conjunctiva

Vascular abnormalities

Haemangioma
- Usually associated with lid and orbital haemangioma (Fig. 10.1).
- Bright red, blanch on pressure.
- Spontaneous haemorrhages occur.
- Spontaneous improvement in infancy.
- Surgical removal may be followed by recurrence.
- Radiotherapy may help.

Lymphohaemangioma
- Mixture of clear fluid and blood-filled cysts.
- Widespread involvement of the face, palate, etc. (Fig. 10.2).
- Spontaneous improvement less frequent.

Sturge–Weber syndrome
- Diffuse conjunctival vascularisation sometimes with larger vessels (Fig. 10.3) (see Chapter 24).

Other conjunctival vascular abnormalities with systemic involvement
- Klippel–Trenaunay–Weber syndrome: skin and bone vascular anomalies.
- Wyburn–Mason syndrome (see Chapter 17):
  - (a) racemose retinal angioma;
  - (b) orbital and intracranial vascular malformations.

Ataxia telangiectasia (Louis–Bar syndrome)
- Autosomal recessive.
- Cerebellar ataxia.
- Immune deficiency.
- Mental and growth regression.
- Telangiectatic conjunctival vessels (Fig. 10.4).

Box 10.1 Conjunctival haemorrhage

- Minor trauma.
- Idiopathic, spontaneous.
- Vascular malformation.
- Thrombocytopenia.
- Leukaemia, etc.
- Haemorrhagic conjunctivitis.
- Hypersensitivity.
- Excessive coughing (pertussis).
- Chronic raised venous pressure.

Treatment is that of the underlying condition. Anomalous vessels may be cauterized. Spontaneous improvement.

Pigmented conjunctival lesions

1. Oculodermal melanocytosis (naevus of Ota):
   (a) ipsilateral skin and mucous membrane pigmentation;
   (b) conjunctiva and subconjunctival pigmentation.
2. Ocular melanosis:
   (a) conjunctival and subconjunctival pigmentation (Fig. 10.5);
   (b) variable slate blue colour;
   (c) malignant change unusual;
   (d) glaucoma may occur.
3. Conjunctival naevi:
   (a) benign conjunctival pigmented tumours (Fig. 10.6);
   (b) usually limbal;
   (c) flat or slightly raised;
   (d) variably pigmented;
   (e) very slow progression;
   (f) treatment by excision for cosmetic reasons.
4. Epibulbar dermoid:
   (a) choristoma, with fat, hair and sebaceous glands;
   (b) occasionally contain other tissue (Fig. 10.7);

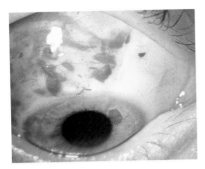

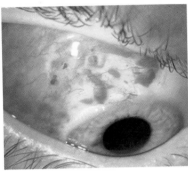

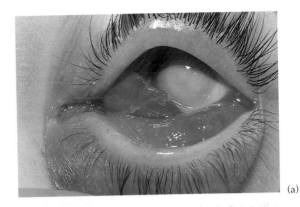

(a)

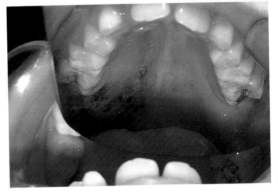

(b)

Fig. 10.1 Conjunctival haemangioma. As a baby this 17-year-old girl had an orbital and lid haemangioma. The subconjunctival vascular abnormality had bled repeatedly and did not respond to surgical excision of the subconjunctival vessels. It became devascularized with low-dose radiotherapy.

Fig. 10.2 (a) This 2-year-old child had an anomalous left eye from birth. At 18 months of age the lids became swollen due to a lymphohaemangioma which also involved the orbit and maxilla. (b) Clear and blood-filled cysts typical of lymphohaemangioma are seen on the palate.

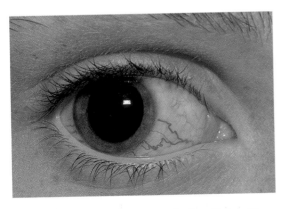

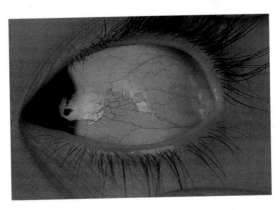

Fig. 10.3 Sturge–Weber syndrome. Conjunctival capillary haemangioma with dilated larger vessels associated with glaucoma.

Fig. 10.4 Ataxia telangiectasia. There is a group of telangiectatic and tortuous vessels in the exposed area of the conjunctiva, especially temporally.

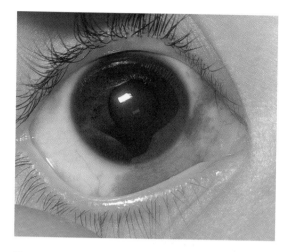

Fig. 10.5 Ocular melanosis. Congenital slate-blue episcleral pigmentation.

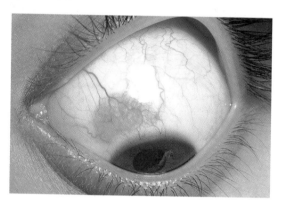

Fig. 10.6 Pigmented cystic compound naevus in the conjunctiva of a 14-year-old boy.

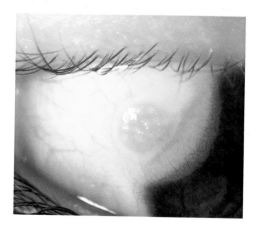

Fig. 10.7 A hairy limbal dermoid.

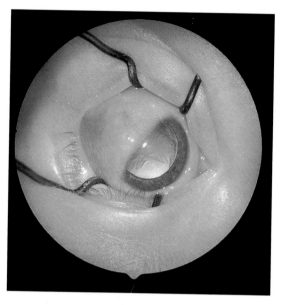

Fig. 10.8 A limbal epibulbar dermoid encroaching on the lateral third of the cornea. Although removed, leaving minimal scarring, the eye had profound amblyopia due to astigmatism.

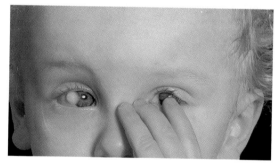

Fig. 10.9 Right limbal dermoid in a child with Goldenhar's syndrome. He also had corneal anaesthesia affecting the left eye particularly and can be seen scratching the cornea at the time when the picture was taken.

(c) posteriorly located epibulbar dermoids may contain more fat and other tissues and are known as dermolipomas;

(d) treatment is by surgical excision, with care being taken to carefully define the posterior extent and to avoid damage to muscles, etc. Associated corneal dermoids may be excised by simple

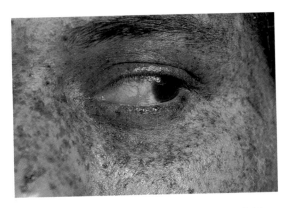

Fig. 10.10 Xeroderma pigmentosa. The widespread skin pigmentation can be seen in this girl of Indian origin. The conjunctiva was affected by multifocal recurrent squamous cell carcinomas.

keratectomy or combined with a free-hand corneal graft (Fig. 10.8);

(e) may be associated with Goldenhar's syndrome (Fig. 10.9).

5 Clear cysts:
   (a) post-traumatic or post-surgical;
   (b) spontaneous;
   (c) cysts of conjunctival glands.
6 Secondary tumours:
   (a) rhabdomyosarcoma;
   (b) retinoblastoma;
   (c) Langerhan's cell histiocystosis;
   (d) juvenile xanthogranuloma;
   (e) leukaemia;
   (f) neurofibromas.

7 Xeroderma pigmentosa:
   (a) autosomal recessive;
   (b) light sensitivity giving pigmentation, telangiectasis;
   (c) basal cell and squamous cell carcinomas, malignant melanomas;
   (d) chronic conjunctivitis;
   (e) conjunctival squamous cell carcinoma and malignant carcinoma (Fig. 10.10);
   (f) treatment by prevention of light exposure, early excision of tumour.
8 pingueculum and pterygium:
   (a) rare in childhood;
   (b) localised drying, i.e. after squint surgery, excision of epibulbar masses.

Box 10.2 Conjunctival scarring

1 Burns.
2 Trauma, i.e. surgical.
3 Infection:
   (a) trachoma;
   (b) chronic conjunctivitis.
4 Avitaminosis A.
5 Post-inflammatory:
   (a) Stevens–Johnson syndrome;
   (b) Richner–Hanhart syndrome (see Chapter 11);
   (c) chronic vernal disease;
   (d) epidermolysis bullosa.
6 Dry eye.
7 Ectodermal dysplasia.
8 Drugs:
   (a) systemic;
   (b) topical (lower fornix, i.e. chronic medication).

11: Cornea

Developmental abnormalities

Because different structures in the anterior segment are subject to common influences, congenital anomalies of the cornea are commonly associated with iris abnormalities and/or glaucoma. Recognizable patterns of clinical presentation are apparent but there is considerable overlap. Anterior segment maldevelopment may be genetically determined with or without systemic features. It may also be the result of toxic insult (i.e. in the fetal alcohol syndrome).

Primary corneal abnormalities

Whole cornea

Megalocornea

Megalocornea is defined as a cornea with a horizontal diameter of more than 13 mm that does not show progressive enlargement. Intraocular pressure is normal as are cell density and corneal thickness. Other features of this bilateral syndrome are arcus juvenilis, mosaic corneal dystrophy, pigment dispersion and cataract and lens dislocation. The refraction is usually low myopia with astigmatism or emmetropia. As a result, visual development is normal. Most commonly this is an X-linked disorder; a gene locus has been identified on the long arm of the X chromosome in the region Xq12–q26, although autosomal recessive and dominant inheritance has also been documented (Fig. 11.1).

Megalocornea may be associated with several systemic disorders including:
- ichthyosis and poikilodermia congenita;
- Aarskog's syndrome — X-linked recessive disorder with short stature, hypertelorism, antimongoloid slant, saddle deformity of the scrotum and syndactyly;
- Marfan's syndrome;
- the megalocornea mental retardation syndrome—

mental retardation, short stature, ataxia and seizures;
- Kneist's syndrome;
- non-ketotic hyperglycaemia.
  Other ocular associations include:
- ectopia lentis et pupillae — autosomal recessive condition with posterior displacement of lens, myopia, cataract, persistent pupillary membrane, retinal detachment;
- congenital miosis;
- Rieger's anomaly;
- albinism;
- Weill–Marchesani syndrome;
- Crouzon's syndrome;
- Marshall–Smith syndrome — failure to thrive, mental retardation and dysmorphia;
- SHORT syndrome — short stature, hyperextensible joints, ocular depression, Rieger's anomaly, teething delay.

Microcornea

Microcornea is an uncommon condition with a cornea less than 10 mm in diameter.

Microphthalmos is defined as an eye with an axial length of greater than two standard deviations below the mean (usually due to a small anterior segment but normal posterior one).

Microcornea may be associated with corneal opacification, vascularisation, anterior segment dysgenesis, cataract, congenital aphakia, coloboma, persistent hyperplastic vitreous (PHPV), retinal dysplasia and ipsilateral facial malformation.

Cornea plana

Cornea plana is defined as a cornea with a curvature of 20–40 D. Keratometry readings of the cornea will be equal to or less than the sclera. The condition may be unilateral or bilateral. Associated ocular conditions include infantile glaucoma, retinal dysplasia,

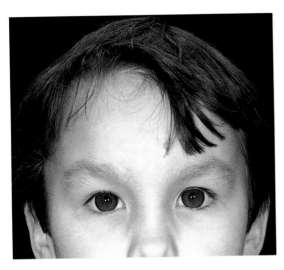

Fig. 11.1 Megalocornea: corrected acuities were normal.

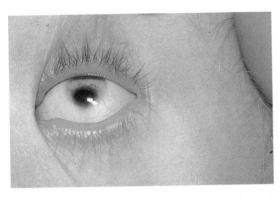

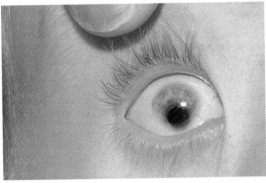

Fig. 11.2 Colobomatous microphthalmos, microcornea and cornea plana.

aniridia, congenital cataracts, ectopia lentis, colobomas, blue sclera and microphthalmos. Refractive errors are usually hyperopic, although myopia and astigmatism occasionally occur. Inheritance is either autosomal dominant or recessive (Fig. 11.2).

Corneal clouding or diffuse opacities
- Congenital glaucoma.
- Sclerocornea.
- Corneal dystrophies (particularly congenital hereditary endothelial dystrophy (CHED) — see p. 85).
- Mucopolysaccharidosis.
- Cystinosis.
- Widespread anterior segment dysgenesis.
- Chemical injury.
- Fetal alcohol syndrome.
- Infective keratitis (see Chapter 5).
- Non-infective keratitis (see below).
- Skin diseases (see below).

Box 11.1 Fetal alcohol syndrome

- Corneal stromal oedema.
- Thickening or loss of Bowman's membrane.
- Sometimes Peter's anomaly.
- Other ocular features of the fetal alcohol syndrome:
  (a) microphthalmos;
  (b) optic nerve hypoplasia;
  (c) strabismus;
  (d) short palpebral fissures;
  (e) epicanthus;
  (f) ptosis.
- Systemic manifestations of the fetal alcohol syndrome:
  (a) mental retardation;
  (b) low birth weight;
  (c) abnormalities of the cardiovascular and skeletal system;
  (d) flat philtrum;
  (e) turned-up nose.

Peripheral corneal opacities
Dermoid
A dermoid consists of collagen connective tissue with epithelium giving it a white solid mass. Epibulbar dermoids may be located in the conjunctiva, sclera, cornea or at the limbus. They may occur as

an isolated anomaly or as part of the ring dermoid syndrome — bilateral 360° dermoids with corneal, limbal, scleral and conjunctival components associated with corneal astigmatism, amblyopia and strabismus.

Sclerocornea

Sclerocornea is a congenital, bilateral, peripheral corneal opacification with vascularization that is often asymmetrical. Fifty per cent of cases are sporadic and 50% are of an autosomal recessive disorder (Fig. 11.3). When isolated it may present with other ocular features including:
- microcornea;
- cornea plana;
- glaucoma;
- angle dysgenesis;
- strabismus;
- nystagmus.

Rarely, it may be associated with systemic abnormalities including:
- spina bifida;
- mental retardation;
- cerebellar abnormalities;
- Hallermann–Streiff syndrome;
- Mieten's syndrome;
- Smith–Lemli–Optiz syndrome;
- osteogenesis imperfecta;
- hereditary osteomychodysplasia — visual acuity in this syndrome is usually good if glaucoma is not associated with it.

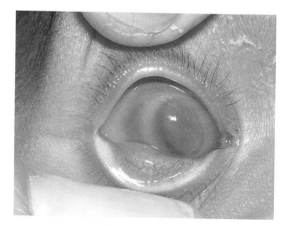

Fig. 11.3 Sclerocornea.

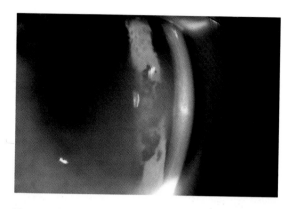

Fig. 11.4 Bilateral Peter's anomaly with peripheral scleralisation of the cornea.

Central corneal opacities

Peter's anomaly

This is usually a bilateral condition with congenital central corneal opacification and clear peripheral corneas. An underlying cataract is frequent. It may be an isolated anomaly or associated with other ocular malformations including:
- glaucoma;
- microcornea;
- microphthalmos;
- cornea plana;
- coloboma;
- mesenchymal dysgenesis of the iris (Fig. 11.4).

It may be part of the Peter's Plus syndrome: a syndrome characterized by short stature, cleft lip or palate, abnormal ears and developmental delay.

Other syndromes in which Peter's anomaly occurs include:
- fetal alcohol syndrome;
- ring 21 chromosomal abnormality;
- partial deletion of the long arm of chromosome 11;
- Warburg's syndrome.

Treatment of Peter's anomaly is aimed at detecting and treating the associated glaucoma as well as clearing the visual axis if possible (Fig. 11.5). However, since the surgical results or penetrating keratoplasty in the treatment of Peter's anomaly are generally poor most authorities agree that only bilateral severe cases should be submitted to kerato-

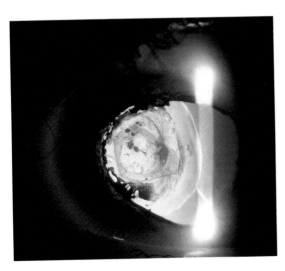

Fig. 11.5 The left eye of this patient with Peter's anomaly has glaucoma which was controlled by a single trabeculectomy. The eye is aphakic with lens cornea adhesion and extensive iris hypoplasia, seen here in retroillumination.

plasty. Optical iridectomy may help those with purely central corneal and lens defects.

Posterior keratoconus

This is a rare syndrome that is binocular, congenital and non-progressive. The anterior corneal curvature is normal but there is an area of stromal thinning on the posterior surface associated with increased curvature. Myopic astigmatism results from it.

Primary angle abnormalities

The posterior limit of Descemet's membrane is demarcated by Schwalbe's ring. Its anterior border may be visible as a narrow, grey–white line known as posterior embryotoxon (Fig. 11.6).

Posterior embryotoxon may be clinically evident in a significant number of otherwise normal eyes. However, developmental abnormalities of the anterior segment may accompany posterior embryotoxon in several important syndromes.

Axenfeld's anomaly

Axenfeld's anomaly consists of posterior embryotoxon in association with iridogoniodysgenesis (iris tissues may be seen adherent to Schwalbe's

ring). It may occur sporadically or be inherited as an autosomal dominant disorder. Fifty per cent of affected patients will develop glaucoma (Fig. 11.7).

Congenital glaucoma

Congenital glaucoma is a form of angle dysgenesis due to failure of development of the normal discontinuity of cells lining the angle.

Alagille's syndrome

This is an autosomal dominantly inherited syndrome with congenital intrahepatic bile duct hypoplasia leading to jaundice. Posterior

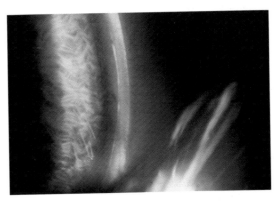

Fig. 11.6 Posterior embryotoxon. This common anomaly can be seen in the slit beam.

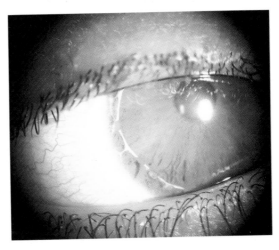

Fig. 11.7 Axenfeld's anomaly—marked posterior embryotoxon to which is attached strands of iris.

embryotoxon is seen in greater than 90% of patients. The fundi are pale and optic disc drusen are present. Other associated anomalies include vertebral butterfly arch malformations, cardiovascular defects, deep-set eyes, hypertelorism and a pointed chin. An associated pigmentory retinopathy may occur due to vitamin A and E deficiencies.

Iris abnormalities associated with posterior embryotoxon

Rieger's anomaly

- Hypoplasia of the anterior iris stroma.
- Iridotrabecular bridges to Schwalbe's line.
- Posterior embryotoxon (Fig. 11.8).
  Other features may include:
- ectropion uvea;
- coloboma of the iris;
- high myopia;
- retinal detachment;
- glaucoma—in at least 60% of cases;
- corneal opacities—usually small and peripheral;
- posterior keratoconus;
- cataracts—usually small, localised cortical opacities; not usually visually significant;
- optic disc anomalies—tilting, myelination.

Rieger's anomaly is usually inherited as autosomal dominant with some 30% of cases being either sporadic or new mutations (Fig. 11.9) .

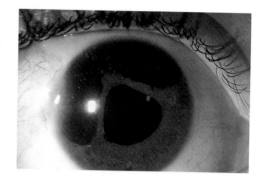

Fig. 11.8 Rieger's syndrome showing iris hypoplasia and polycoria.

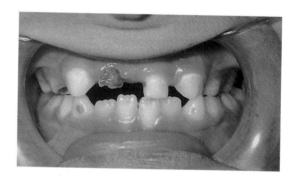

Fig. 11.9 Rieger's anomaly showing the dental abnormalities, widely spaced conical teeth and partial anadontia. There is also caries.

> ### Box 11.2 Rieger's syndrome
>
> Rieger's syndrome consists of the ocular features of Rieger's anomaly with somatic features including:
> - maxillary hypoplasia;
> - short philtrum;
> - dental anomalies — small, widely space cone-shaped teeth, partial anodontia;
> - umbilical and inguinal hernias;
> - hypospadias;
> - isolated growth hormone deficiencies;
> - cardiac valvular disease.
>
> Abnormalities of chromosome 6 as well as deletions of chromosome 13 (4q25–4q27) have been associated with this syndrome. It is inherited as an autosomal dominant trait syndrome. Twenty-five to fifty per cent of affected individuals will develop glaucoma (Fig. 11.9).

Other syndromes associated with anterior segment maldevelopment include the following.

- *Michel's syndrome.* This is an autosomal recessive syndrome in which cleft lip and palate are associated with epicanthus, telecanthus, ptosis, reduced intelligence, telangiectatic conjunctival vessels, peripheral corneal opacities and iridocorneal adhesions.
- *Oculo-dento-digital dysplasia.* This is an autosomal dominant syndrome associated with microphthalmos, iris hypoplasia, persistent pupillary membranes, small nose, hypoplastic alae, narrow and short palpebral fissures, telecanthus, epicanthus, sparse eyebrows, dental enamel hypoplasia and camptodactyly or syndactyly of the ulnar two or three digits. Abnormal angles with iridodysgenesis predispose these patients to develop glaucoma.

Acquired corneal abnormalities in childhood

Keratitis

Allergic
See Chapter 6.

Infection
See Chapter 6.

Exposure keratitis

Exposure keratitis is a result of inadequate lubrication and protection for the corneal epithelium. Damage is usually limited to the corneal epithelium but when cases are complicated with secondary bacterial infections, perforation of the cornea may occur (Fig. 11.10).

Exposure keratitis may come about as the result of the following.

• Eyelid abnormalities — these result in poor tear film distribution.

• Disorders of the lacrimal gland — resulting in decreased tear production.

• Central nervous system disease—interferes with neural supply of the lacrimal system and/or cornea.

• Orbital disease — produces proptosis with poor lid closure.

• Fifth and/or seventh nerve palsies — by far the most difficult patients to manage are those with combined fifth and seventh cranial nerve palsies. Patients should be treated with frequent tear

---

Box 11.3 Non-infective keratitis

1 Trauma:
(a) acute, especially with embedded foreign bodies;
(b) chronic, i.e. trichiasis, repeated trauma in anaesthetic corneas.
2 Hypoxia:
(a) prolonged contact lens wear;
(b) usually apical.
3 Ischaemia:
(a) rare in childhood;
(b) coagulation vasculopathies, autoimmune disease, etc.
4 Chemical and physical irritants:
(a) acid or alkaline burns;
(b) post-irradiation, compounded by dry eye.
5 Dry eye: keratitis initially non-infective but infection soon intervenes.
6 Avitaminosis A.
7 Associated with non-infective inflammatory disease:
(a) Stevens–Johnson;
(b) staphylococcal hypersensitivity;
(c) vernal disease.
8 Tyrosinaemia type II (Richner–Hanhart syndrome):
(a) amoeboid or other apical keratitis;
(b) skin lesions on pressure points of hands and feet;
(c) treatable by dietary means.

---

replacements, ointments at night time, bandage contact lenses, moisture chambers and antibiotics when secondary infections occur (Fig. 11.11).

Trauma

(See Chapter 25.) A wide variety of traumatic injuries to the cornea may occur in childhood. These include the following.

• Non-accidental injury — in child abuse one may see corneal epithelial abrasion, penetrating and perforating injuries of the cornea associated with hyphaema.

• Forceps injury — cause ruptures of Descemet's membrane, usually in a vertical direction; myopia and astigmatism may lead to amblyopia.

• Chemical injuries — both acid and alkali burns may occur in children (Fig. 11.12).

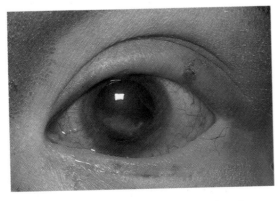

Fig. 11.10 Keratitis resulting from a combination of exposure, drying and the direct effects of irradiation for orbital rhabdomyosarcoma.

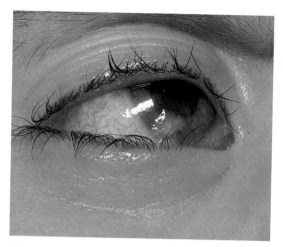

Fig. 11.11 Dry and exposed eye giving rise to keratitis in a patient with seventh nerve palsy associated with the CHARGE syndrome.

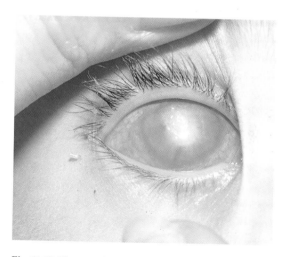

Fig. 11.12 Non-accidental chemical injury to the eye. This child suddenly developed a profoundly severe keratitis in one eye on the day that his mother's boyfriend left home. Although never proven the situation was highly suggestive.

Cogan's syndrome

This syndrome consists of interstitial keratitis and audiovestibular dysfunction. The interstitial keratitis may be associated with vascularization and uveitis. Eighth nerve involvement may precede or follow corneal involvement. The cause is unknown.

Vitamin A deficiency and measles

Avitaminosis A may produce thickening of the corneal epithelium, keratization of the epithelium and diffuse corneal opacification. Secondary pannus and corneal vascularization can occur. In addition to corneal pathology, white foamy lesions of the temporal conjunctiva are seen — these are called Bitot's spots (see Chapter 10).

When vitamin A deficiency is accompanied by malnourishment and protein deficiency an acute liquefactive necrosis of the cornea may occur. Predisposing risk factors for this include infection with measles and herpes simplex and the use of traditional eye medicines.

Acute keratomalacia associated with avitaminosis is a medical emergency. Treatment should include a high-protein and calorie diet with vitamin A replacement.

Ectodermal dysplasia

Ectodermal dysplasia is a very rare syndrome inherited as either an X-linked or autosomal recessive condition. It is characterized by abnormal eccrine glands, wispy or absent hair and abnormal teeth or nails (Fig. 11.13).

Two main forms of this syndrome are seen as either hidrotic or hypohidrotic. Corneal changes within this syndrome include corneal cysts, opacities, pannus formation, dry eye syndrome with secondary corneal changes and infectious keratitis.

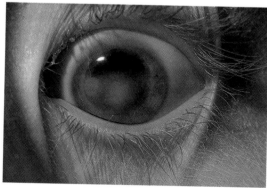

Fig. 11.13 Ectodermal dysplasia with superficial corneal opacities.

Epidermolysis bullosa (EB)

In dystrophic EB there are absent anchoring fibrils at the conjunctival dermo–epidermal junction and abnormal attachment complexes between corneal epithelium and basement membrane. Nevertheless, corneal abnormalities are surprisingly infrequent but may include:

- limbal broadening;
- corneal reticular opacity;
- symblepharon (Fig. 11.14).

Ichthyosis

The ichthyosiform dermatoses are a group of disorders characterized by scaling. In their extreme congenital forms affected individuals may die as a result of uncontrolled skin infections. Different ichthyosiform dermatoses include the following.

- Ichthyosis vulgaris—autosomal dominant trait—no eye problems.
- X-linked ichthyosis—scaling of scalp, face, neck, abdomen and limbs—thickening of corneal nerves with band keratopathy. Superficial epithelial corneal scarring may occur. Posterior corneal opacities are less common.
- Lamellar ichthyosis and ichthyosis linearis—severe autosomal recessive disorders—ectropion and keratoconjunctivitis, mainly secondary to exposure, occur.
- Epidermolytic hyperkeratoses and erythrokeratoderma variabilis—autosomal dominant conditions—corneal involvement (Fig. 11.15).

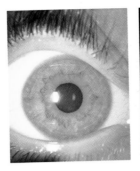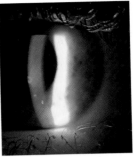

Fig. 11.15 Ichthyosis with superficial corneal lesions.

Other syndromes with ichthyosis include:

- Sjögren–Larssen syndrome;
- Netherton's syndrome;
- Refsum's syndrome;
- chondrodysplasia punctata;
- IBIDS syndrome;
- KIDS syndrome.

Corneal anaesthesia and hypoaesthesia

Lack of corneal sensation may give rise to a keratitis. This is often termed neurotrophic keratitis, although the major aetiological factors are drying of the tear film with reduced blinking and repetitive corneal trauma rather than the absence of a neurotrophic factor for the cornea.

Defective corneal sensation can be secondary to fifth nerve damage associated with:

- herpes zoster;
- trauma;
- intracranial tumours;
- herpes simplex;
- oculofacial syndromes;
- Goldenhar's syndrome;
- leprosy;
- carbon disulphide or hydrogen sulphide poisoning;
- Riley–Day syndrome;
- MURCS syndrome (Fig. 11.16).

Patients develop recurrent erosions that are difficult to manage and may become secondarily infected. Cases with lagophthalmos or defective tears are particularly difficult to treat. This combination is seen in the Riley–Day syndrome (Fig. 11.17), leprosy and some brainstem tumours.

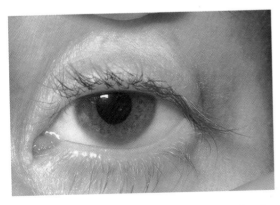

Fig. 11.14 EB showing expanded limbus and peripheral pannus.

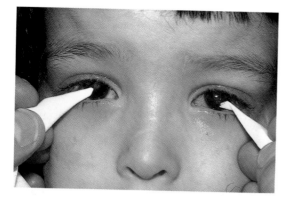

Fig. 11.16 Profound corneal anaesthesia which allows the eye to be touched and keratitis to occur without pain.

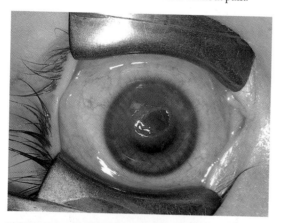

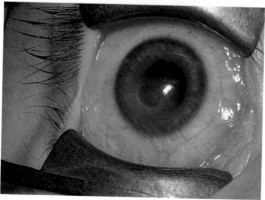

Fig. 11.17 Riley–Day syndrome. This child had a combination of anaesthetic corneas and dry eyes that had been treated for several months by topical wetting agents without success. He responded well to a bilateral tarsorrhaphy and lubricant ointment. Later, punctal occlusion allowed even wetting of his eyes and the tarsorrhaphies were undone.

Treatment consists of intensive lubrication with artificial tears and ointment. Intermittent topical antibiotics may be necessary to prevent secondary bacterial infection. If lagophthalmos occurs the lids should be patched at night whilst the patient is sleeping or a tarsorrhaphy completed.

Keratoconus

Keratoconus is an ectatic dystrophy of the cornea resulting in central or paracentral thinning, usually affecting patients after the first decade of life (Fig. 11.18). The cause is unknown although trauma may play an important role. Inheritance is not predictable but in certain families there is a definite family history. Most cases are sporadic.

The symptoms of keratoconus are primarily related to its secondary visual impairment; corneal thinning leads to increasing amounts of astigmatism which is irregular and usually requires contact lens correction (Fig. 11.19). As the disorder progresses, stretching of Descemet's membrane results in a failure of corneal dehydration, resulting in a condition known as acute hydrops (Fig. 11.20). In this condition blurred vision caused by corneal oedema may be accompanied by severe pain. This will resolve spontaneously leaving variable corneal

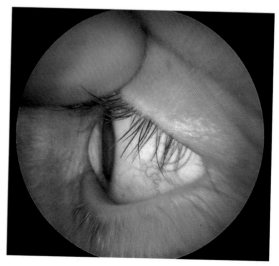

Fig. 11.18 Keratoconus. Side view showing the conical cornea and the outward bowing of the lower lid (Munson's signs).

- Crouzon's disease;
- Down's syndrome;
- Ehlers–Danlos syndrome;
- Laurence–Moon–Biedl syndrome;
- Marfan's syndrome;
- mitral valve prolapse;
- Noonan's syndrome;
- osteogenesis imperfecta;
- Raynaud's syndrome;
- syndactyly;
- exoderma pigmentosum;
- Leber's congenital amaurosis (and other congenital cone–rod dystrophies).

Keratoglobus

Unlike keratoconus, the stromal thinning in keratoglobus occurs in the centre of the cornea. This may occur in conjunction with keratoconus or as a separate disorder. Keratoglobus may be associated with:

- blue sclerae;
- joint hyperextensibility, deafness and mottled teeth;
- the Rubinstein–Taybi syndrome (Fig. 11.21).

Metabolic diseases involving the cornea

Metabolic diseases may affect the cornea in any of its layers.

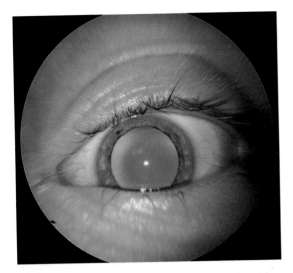

Fig. 11.19 Keratoconus. The retinoscopic reflex in keratoconus is abnormal with no clear end-point.

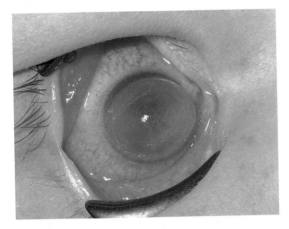

Fig. 11.20 Acute hydrops in a child with Down's syndrome.

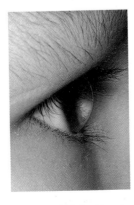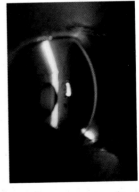

Fig. 11.21 X-linked keratoglobus. On the left it is possible to see into the iridocorneal angle by looking laterally at the eye without using a gonioscope.

scarring. Surgical intervention is not recommended during this acute episode.

Most keratoconus can be managed conservatively with contact lenses but penetrating keratoplasty may be necessary in severe cases.

Keratoconus may be associated with the following systemic conditions:

- Apert's syndrome;
- atopy;
- brachydactyly;

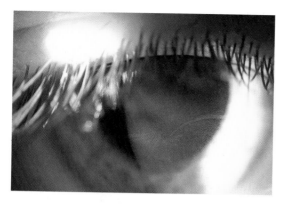

Fig. 11.22 Amiodarone keratopathy. It is unusual for these patients to have a significant visual defect. The most common abnormality is a mild whorl-like opacity as seen in the centre of this photograph.

Epithelial disorders

The corneal epithelium may be stained by toxins or be involved in some metabolic diseases.
• Chloroquine diphosphate and hydroxychloroquine sulphate—whorl-like opacities.
• Amiodarone — vortex pattern, fine punctate opacity (Fig. 11.22).

Subepithelial disorders

Acrodermatitis enteropathica is associated with radial subepithelial lines in the superior portion of the cornea. These are whorl-like. Keratomalacia may occur.

Other symptoms include dystrophic fingernails and gastrointestinal disturbance, producing diarrhoea and poor growth.

Zinc dietary supplements are indicated.

Stromal

In cystinosis, a defect of lysosomal transport, accumulation of cystine occurs in lysosomes. The corneal crystals in cystinosis are mainly in the anterior stroma but they may also produce corneal thickening and be associated with reduced corneal sensitivity, superficial punctate keratopathy and recurrent erosions (Fig. 11.23).

Other associated findings in cystinosis include growth retardation, renal failure, decreased skin and hair pigmentation, and pigmentory retinopa-

thy. An infantile form causes renal failure with early death. An adult form has no renal involvement and is limited to corneal manifestations. An intermediate adolescent form resembles the infantile form but without growth retardation and skin changes.

Cysteamine treatment may be beneficial. Penetrating keratoplasty may be indicated in patients with severe visual loss.

Descemet's membrane

Wilson's disease is an inherited disorder of copper metabolism in which low levels of copper-transporting protein accompany low serum and high tissue levels of copper. The gene appears to be similar to Menkes gene at 3q14.3. The cornea frequently develops staining of the peripheral Descemet's membrane, most marked in the 12 and 6 o'clock positions (Fig. 11.24). This may not be appreciated initially without gonioscopy.

Associated findings include:
• basal ganglia degeneration with tremor;
• choreoathetosis;
• neuropsychiatric changes;
• renal tubular staining with aminoaciduria;
• nodular cirrhosis.

Rarely, in Wilson's disease, a sunflower cataract may be seen (see Chapter 14). Treatment is with penicillamine which may not always be effective, and liver transplantation may be necessary.

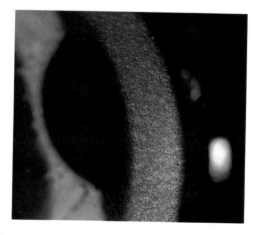

Fig. 11.23 Cystinosis. Corneal crystals can be seen by slit lamp microscopy. The children are often blond, fair-skinned and very photophobic.

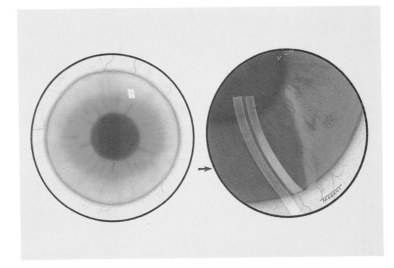

Fig. 11.24 Wilson's disease. The brown deposits are most prominent in the 6 and 12 o'clock positions and consist of depositions of brown–green copper-containing substance in the peripheral parts of Descemet's membrane. Gonioscopy may be necessary for visualization.

Box 11.4 Corneal crystals

Crystal-like corneal deposits occur in the following:
1 cystinosis;
2 crystalline corneal dystrophy (Schnyder's dystrophy);
3 lecithin cholesterol acyltransferase (LCAT) disease;
4 uric acid crystals;
5 granular dystrophy and Bietti's marginal dystrophy;
6 multiple myeloma; monoclonal gammopathies;
7 calcium deposition;
8 dieffenbachia plant keratoconjunctivitis;
9 a syndrome of corneal crystals, myopathy and nephropathy;
10 tyrosinaemia type II.

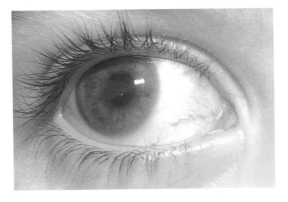

Fig. 11.25 Band keratopathy in a patient with Still's disease.

Band keratopathy

Band keratopathy results from the infiltration of calcium within Bowman's membrane. This usually comes about as the result of chronic inflammation or systemic disease. The deposition occurs primarily in the interpalpebral condition.

Systemic conditions known to be associated with band keratopathy include sarcoidosis, parathyroid disease and multiple myeloma.

Chronic ocular inflammation is also associated with band keratopathy — most commonly juvenile rheumatoid arthritis, Still's disease and sarcoidosis (Fig. 11.25).

Treatment with topical chelating agents may be effective. Band keratopathy often occurs in association with end-stage phthisis bulbi.

Lecithin cholesterol acyltransferase (LCAT) deficiency

LCAT deficiency is an autosomal recessive condition that produces central corneal haze in homozygotes and premature arcus senilis in heterozygotes.

Systemic findings associated with it may include renal failure, anaemia and hyperlipidaemia.

Corneal arcus

Arcus lipoides is due to a deposition of a variety of phospholipids, low-density lipoproteins and triglycerides in the peripheral stromal tissue. Arcus appears in young patients in association with:
• familial hypercholesterolaemia (Friederickson's type II) (Fig. 11.26);
• familial hyperlipoproteinaemia (type III);
• adjacent to corneal disease such as vernal keratopathy or herpes simplex infection (Fig. 11.27);
• primary lipoidal degeneration of the corneas.
Arcus may occur in healthy corneas in a person with normal plasma lipids.

Box 11.5   Blue sclera

Hereditary conditions that cause a defect in mesodermal structures will produce a blue sclera, probably as a result of thinning. This may be seen in association with:
• osteogenesis imperfecta;
• Ehlers–Danlos syndrome;
• Hallermann–Strieff syndrome;
• Marfan's syndrome;
• brittle corneas;
• ectodermal dysplasia.
In infancy many normal children have bluish corneas unassociated with any pathology.

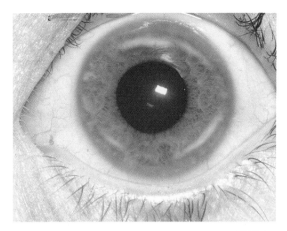

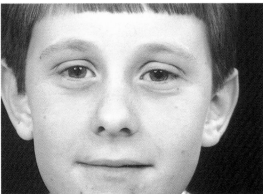

Fig. 11.27 Corneal arcus remaining in a child who had severe vernal catarrh.

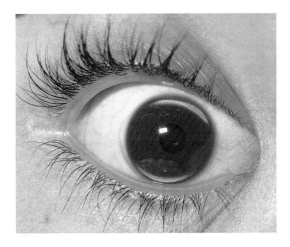

Fig. 11.26 Corneal arcus in a patient with hyperlipidaemia.

Hyphaema and corneal blood staining

Blood staining of the cornea is an important and devastating complication of hyphaema. Generally, duration of hyphaema, degree of intraocular pressure and presence of corneal damage are all important prognostic factors in determining whether a hyphaema will be followed by corneal blood staining. Rebleeding during the post-injury period is especially a poor prognostic sign. No medications that interfere with normal clotting mechanisms should be given for analgesia in the child with a hyphaema. Corneal blood staining is usually associated with decreased visual acuity and occasionally amblyopia. Rarely, penetrating keratoplasty may be necessary to treat it (see Chapter 25).

Multiple endocrine neoplasia (MEN)

There are three main syndromes in which tumours occur in a variety of endocrine organs at a young age. MEN type IIb is most important to the ophthalmologist. Patients exhibit a marfanoid habitus, full fleshy lips, nodular neuromas on the tip and edges of the tongue and margins of eyelids, pes cavus, constipation and peroneal muscular atrophy. Prominent corneal nerves within an otherwise normal cornea are an important diagnostic feature. Because of a very high incidence of thyroid medullary carcinoma in MEN IIb, prophylactic thyroidectomy may be recommended in childhood. Phaeochromocytoma may be associated (Fig. 11.28).

Box 11.6 Enlarged corneal nerves

- MEN IIb.
- Dystrophies: Fuchs', keratoconus.
- Buphthalmos.
- Inflammatory disease—leprosy.
- Refsum's disease.
- Ichthyosis.
- Neurofibromatosis.

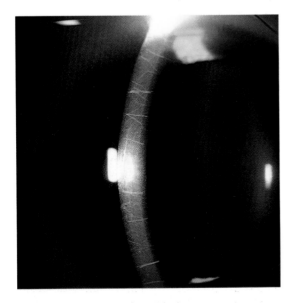

Fig. 11.28 MEN type IIb. Thickened corneal nerves can be seen crossing even the axial area of the cornea.

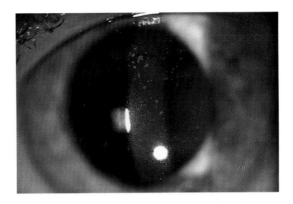

Fig. 11.29 Map, dot and fingerprint dystrophy.

Corneal dystrophies

Corneal dystrophies are inherited conditions, and are usually bilateral and symmetrical. Dystrophies are to be distinguished from corneal degenerations that are secondary non-genetic processes resulting from ageing or previous corneal inflammation.

- *Map, dot, fingerprint; Cogan's microcystic, basement membrane dystrophy.* Autosomal dominant, fingerprint-looking lines just below the epithelium, rarely visually significant. Not associated with systemic disorders. The only symptomatic problem arises from recurrent erosions (Fig. 11.29).
- *Juvenile epithelial dystrophy; Meesman–Wilke's dystrophy.* Autosomal dominant inheritance with incomplete penetrance. Tiny epithelial vesicles. Symptoms of ocular irritation and photophobia due to recurrent erosions. Vision rarely affected. Contact lenses may be indicated for persistent erosion.
- *Reis–Bucklers' dystrophy.* Autosomal dominant inheritance presenting in infancy. Recurrent attacks of photophobia, pain and redness. Microscopic subepithelial protrusions caused by abnormal material at the level of Bowman's membrane. Corneal sensation may be reduced. Visual impairment occurs in the third to fourth decade. Keratoplasty may be necessary (Fig. 11.30).
- *Granular dystrophy; Groenow type I.* Autosomal dominant inheritance. Constant expressivity in all generations. Linked to chromosome 5q. Granular-appearing corneal opacities initially superficial to Bowman's membrane but progress into stroma.

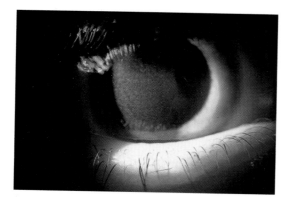

Fig. 11.30 Reis–Buckler's dystrophy showing the irregular corneal surface with subepithelial opacity.

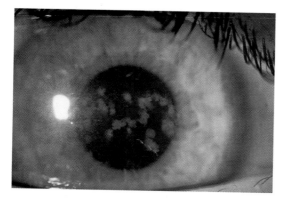

Fig. 11.31 Macular dystrophy showing corneal stromal haziness between the whitish opacity.

Rarely visually significant in childhood. May require penetrating keratoplasty in fifth or sixth decade.

• *Lattice dystrophy; Haab–Biber–Dimer's dystrophy.* Autosomal dominant condition, linked to chromosome 5q. Frequently asymmetrical. Deposition of amyloid in cornea. Lattice lines usually not apparent until adulthood. Penetrating keratoplasty may be necessary in early adulthood. Occasionally associated with systemic amyloidosis and progressive cranial and peripheral nerve palsies.

• *Macular dystrophy; Groenow type II.* Autosomal recessive trait. Rarely symptomatic in childhood. Corneal thickness and stromal haze increases with age. Penetrating keratoplasty not usually required until adulthood (Fig. 11.31).

• *Central crystalline dystrophy; Schnyder.* Autosomal dominant with variable expressivity. Central disc-like opacification with or without cholesterol crystal deposition. Associated with arcus lipoides. Diffuse stromal haze occurs in adulthood requiring penetrating keratoplasty.

• *Dermochondrial corneal dystrophy.* Rare, central anterior dystrophy associated with cataract, skin nodules and limb deformities.

• *Posterior polymorphous dystrophy; Schlichting.* Autosomal dominant. Asymmetrical and slowly progressive. Apparent even in young children as a

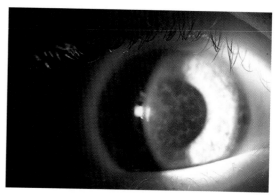

Fig. 11.32 Polymorphus dystrophy. Direct illumination showing geographical opacities.

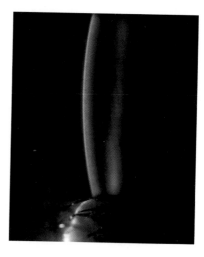

Fig. 11.33 CHED showing opaque and thickened cornea on slit illumination.

ring opacity deep in the cornea at the level of Descemet's membrane. May be associated with anterior chamber cleavage abnormalities and glaucoma. Not usually visually symptomatic (Fig. 11.32).

• *CHED; Maumenee.* Autosomal dominant or recessive inheritance. Present at birth. Diffuse avascular ground-glass bluish-white haziness of the cornea. Increased corneal thickness. May improve with time and not require penetrating keratoplasty (Fig. 11.33).

12: Lacrimal System

Congenital anomalies

1 Lacrimal gland — congenital absence. It is rare and usually associated with other eye and conjunctival abnormalities including Fraser's syndrome and the lacrimo-auriculo-dento-digital syndrome (LADD).
2 Alacrima. Congenital lack of secretion of tears in mild degree is common. It occurs either in an isolated form or associated with familial dysautonomia. Complications include corneal damage and discomfort.
3 Ectopic lacrimal gland—forming an orbital mass.
4 Lacrimal tissue (normally non-functioning) within dermoid cysts.
5 Lacrimal fistulas, in which there is an exit of tears directly via a fistula through the skin.
6 Crocodile tears. This occurs as a consequence of aberrant innervation between the fifth and seventh cranial nerves. Patients' eyes water when eating, often associated with Duane's syndrome.

Dry eyes

Tears normally have a three-layered structure.
1 An oily 'lipid' layer which reduces evaporation, provides a perfect optical surface and stabilizes the tear surface. The lipid is produced in the meibomian glands.
2 The aqueous layer from the lacrimal glands.
3 A mucous layer from conjunctival glands.
- Tear mucin deficiency:
  (a) trachoma;
  (b) Stevens–Johnson syndrome.
- Tear lipid layer deficiency:
  (a) blepharitis;
  (b) meibomianitis;
  (c) meibomian gland loss secondary to disease or irradiation.

- Tear aqueous deficiency (keratoconjunctivitis sicca):
  (a) congenital alacrima;
  (b) defective reflex tearing;
  (c) localised drying — defective blinking or corneal cover;
  (d) a syndrome of familial glucocorticoid deficiency with achalasia of the cardia;
  (e) ectodermal dysplasia;
  (f) with craniofacial malformations, i.e. Goldenhar's syndrome, craniosynostosis;
  (g) multiple endocrine neoplasia type IIb;
  (h) familial dysautonomia (Riley–Day syndrome)
     (i) Ashkenazi-Jewish parentage
     (ii) autonomic disturbances
     (iii) sensory neuropathy
     (iv) lack of fungiform papillae on tongue
     (v) reduced tearing
     (vi) corneal hypoaesthesia (Fig. 12.1)
     (vii) optic neuropathy;
  (i) Sjögren's syndrome. Dry eyes, mouth and other mucous membranes associated with rheumatoid arthritis or autoimmune disease.

Treatment of dry eyes
1 Treatment of the cause:
  (a) vitamin A deficiency;
  (b) poor corneal cover;
  (c) reduction of excessive tear loss
     (i) an avoidance of dry atmospheres
     (ii) use of hydrophilic contact lenses
     (iii) punctal occlusion
     (iv) moisture chambers.
2 Reduction of tear loss:
  (a) reduction of wetted area—by tarsorrhaphy;
  (b) reduction of evaporation by increasing atmospheric humidity.
3 Artificial tears, i.e. polyvinyl alcohol, methyl cellulose or simple eye ointment.

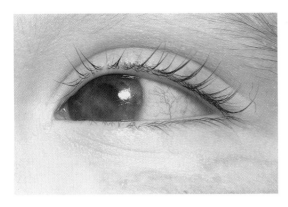

Fig. 12.1 Riley–Day syndrome showing dry eye with corneal hypoaesthesia and severe corneal ulceration and vascularization.

Dacryoadenitis

This is usually associated with a systemic infection (mumps, infectious mononucleosis, herpes zoster, histoplasmosis or gonococcal) or sarcoidosis. There is tenderness and swelling over the lacrimal gland together with a systemic upset and fever. Computerized tomography (CT) scanning demonstrates enlargement and can be useful to exclude associated abnormalities, i.e. leukaemic infiltration or tumour.

Lacrimal drainage system

Congenital punctal and canalicular abnormalities

If the lacrimal canaliculi fail to develop or perforate completely they are difficult to treat in infancy or early childhood. Absence of the upper canaliculus does not usually cause any symptoms, and if just the lower canaliculus is absent, symptoms may not be severe. If both canaliculae are affected the child will have a watering, but not usually sticky, eye. Occasionally, just the punctum is occluded and this may be opened with a punctum dilator and the nasolacrimal system must be intubated. Dacryocystorhinostomy (DCR), together with Lester–Jones tube insertion, is applicable in older children only.

Nasolacrimal fistulas

These are common and occur either as a result of incision of a lacrimal sac abscess or as a congenital anomaly. They can be excised after careful delineation of the canaliculi with dacryocystography or a probe at the time of surgery. Since there is sometimes an associated nasolacrimal duct obstruction this must be probed or a DCR carried out (Fig. 12.2).

Congenital nasolacrimal duct obstruction

1 Isolated.
2 With EEC syndrome — *e*ctodactyly, *e*ctodermal dysplasia, *c*lefting.
3 Craniofacial abnormalities.
4 Down's syndrome.
5 The lacrimal-auriculo-dento-digital syndrome.
6 The CHARGE association (see p. 160).
7 Midfacial defects.

Signs and symptoms
Recurrent watering, discharge and repeated infections indicate nasolacrimal duct obstruction. The eye is not usually significantly red and is never photophobic or uncomfortable. A mucocoele occurs when mucus and/or pus build up in an enlarged sac and can be diagnosed by expressing mucus or mucopus through the punctae by pressure on the lacrimal sac.

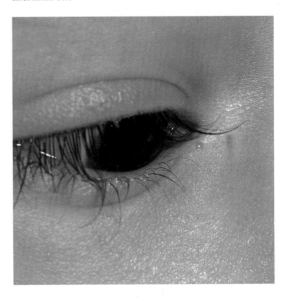

Fig. 12.2 Congenital fistula of the nasolacrimal system. The fistula can be seen as a tiny mark below the medial canthus.

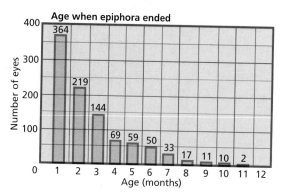

Fig. 12.3 The age when epiphora ended from a large cohort study over the first months of life. It can be seen that only a small proportion of patients with epiphora from congenital nasolacrimal duct obstruction are still symptomatic after 8 months, and the improvement continues. (Courtesy of Dr C.J. MacEwan, with permission.)

Management

1 Since most cases improve spontaneously (Fig. 12.3) treatment is usually expectant unless symptoms are severe.
2 Massage. The mother is taught to massage firmly over the lacrimal sac.

3 Treatment of acute infection with antibiotic drops which should be used only in short courses, i.e. chloromycetin, tobramycin or sulphacetamide four times a day for 5 days only. If the child is still symptomatic between the age of 9 and 12 months then a syringing and probing procedure can be carried out. This is usually done under general anaesthetic.

The technique of syringing and probing

The anaesthetized patient is intubated and a throat pack inserted or a laryngeal mask is used.

The nose is inspected, in particular looking at the inferior turbinate: if this is very large or turned in on itself it can be 'fractured'.

The punctum, usually the upper punctum, is identified and if necessary dilated to accept a lacrimal cannula.

A syringe is loaded with normal saline and the lacrimal cannula on it is inserted in a three-stage process.

1 Vertically through the first 1 mm part of the canaliculus.
2 The lacrimal cannula is gently pushed horizontally through the canaliculus and common canaliculus whilst maintaining some tension on the lid. The cannula must not be forced otherwise a fistula or false passage may occur. When it enters the lacrimal sac, the cannula can be felt to touch bone without causing tension on the lower lid.

It is then rotated downwards and saline syringed. If saline regurgitates through the upper canaliculus, the punctum or canaliculus is occluded either with a cotton wool bud or with a punctum dilator. The increased pressure in the sac causes it to swell and it can be felt in the inner canthus. A patent nasolacrimal duct can be diagnosed by the presence of saline on the throat pack (staining the saline with fluorescein may aid in its identification).

If the nasolacrimal duct is obstructed at its lower end then a probe is carefully inserted in a similar way to that technique used for the cannula, and passed through the nasolacrimal duct breaking down the obstruction. Significant force is not usually necessary. If only a very small size probe is passed at first, it is common practice to use a larger one subsequently.

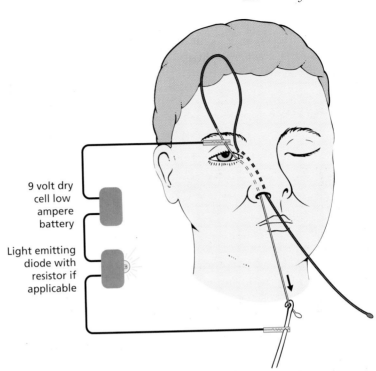

Fig. 12.4 Silicone tube intubation of the nasolacrimal system can be facilitated by location of the Crawford's tube probe under the inferior turbinate by the use of a low-amperage electrical circuit.

9 volt dry cell low ampere battery

Light emitting diode with resistor if applicable

If the nasolacrimal duct is patent then it is assumed that the cause of the watering is due to non-obstructive factors, i.e. swollen nasolacrimal duct mucosa, and this is likely to improve with age. The parents are told beforehand that the procedure is likely to be 80% successful. If an obstruction is found higher up the nasolacrimal duct then a dacryocystorhinostomy is usually necessary.

If a probing has been carried out and the symptoms return it is repeated once, and if the second procedure is unsuccessful, then nasolacrimal duct intubation (Fig. 12.4) is carried out. If that is not successful then dacryocystorhinostomy may be necessary.

Congenital dacryocystocoele

This is also known as amniotocoele, mucocoele or a lacrimal sac cyst. This presents in the neonatal period with a bluish distended lacrimal sac that is not pulsating (in contradistinction to a meningocoele) and it is not inflamed. Some resolve sponta-

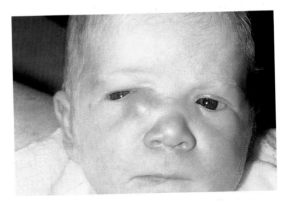

Fig. 12.5 Congenital dacryocystocoele.

neously and others may require massage or probing (Fig. 12.5).

Acquired nasolacrimal duct obstruction

This occurs in diseases of the nose or paranasal

sinuses and is associated with chronic rhinitis. Acquired obstruction may occur with tumours, fibrous dysplasia, craniometaphyseal dysplasia or other bony dysplasias.

Dacryocystitis

Acute

This occurs associated with nasolacrimal duct obstruction, with pain, redness and swelling around the lacrimal sac which may become fluctuant, a systemic upset and a fever.

Management
• Cultures of the conjunctival sac after expression of pus (if possible). Blood culture if the patient is ill.
• Probing is not carried out in the acute phase.
• For acute cases, systemic antibiotics as in preseptal cellulitis (see Chapter 5).
• Incision of the abscess with a wide bore needle is carried out after the acute phase if a fluctuant mass remains.

Chronic

This occurs when the nasolacrimal duct is obstructed. There is tearing and a mucopurulent discharge. Treatment is by massage to express the discharge, topical antibiotic drops and syringing and probing.

Box 12.3 The watering (tearing) eye

1 Nasolacrimal duct obstruction — epiphora, discharge, no redness, no grittiness.
2 Subtarsal or corneal foreign body — watering, grittiness, localized redness, localized fluorescein staining, no discharge.
3 Conjunctivitis — redness, discharge, watering, itchy if allergic.
4 Glaucoma—photophobia, watering, redness only if very severe, no discharge.
5 Crocodile tears — watering which occurs with eating.
6 Contact lens related epiphora — poor fit contact lens, watering and foreign body sensation, giant papillary conjunctivitis.
7 Associated with photophobia—see Chapter 4.

13: Uvea

The uvea consists of the iris, ciliary body and choroid, which are all vascular and heavily pigmented. The uvea has many functions:
• the pupil acts as a variable aperture which is driven by the constrictor and dilator muscles of the iris;
• the pigment of all layers reduces the amount of unnecessary reflected light within the eye and reduces the amount of light coming through the iris;
• the ciliary body secretes aqueous;
• the ciliary muscle and zonule suspends the lens and causes accommodation;
• the choroid supplies nutrients for the outer retinal layers.

At birth the uveal tract is well developed but a pupillary membrane may be present. The ciliary muscle is incomplete and the pars plana is not differentiated until about 1 year of age. Final ciliary body and pars plana length is achieved by 2 years.

Albinism

Albinism is a condition in which there is an abnormality within pigment cells, especially in the eyes and in the skin. The central visual system is also affected. Two main forms occur.
1 Ocular albinism (OA):
  (a) OA1 X-linked OA;
  (b) autosomal recessive OA (AROA).
2 Oculocutaneous albinism (OCA):
  (a) OCA1 tyrosinase deficient OCA;
  (b) OCA2 tyrosinase positive OCA;
  (c) OCA3;
  (d) autosomal dominant OCA (ADOCA).
Albinism may also be associated with systemic disease.

All forms of albinism have common features.
1 Reduced visual acuity and contrast sensitivity:

(a) defective fundus pigmentation;
(b) foveal hypoplasia (Fig. 13.1);
(c) other factors;
(d) nystagmus;
(e) refractive errors;
(f) amblyopia.
2 Nystagmus. The onset may be after a few months of life and the nystagmus is often pendular or compound.
3 Strabismus:
  (a) esotropia;
  (b) exotropia;
  (c) rudimentary binocular vision.
4 Iris translucency. This varies from the mild whose irises are brown or blue (Fig. 13.2), to the pink or blue/pink (Fig. 13.3) in those whose irises are very lightly pigmented.
5 Photophobia. This results from the excessive light transmitted through the translucent irides. This excessive light transmission accounts for why the B wave on the electroretinograph (ERG) is increased in some patients.
6 Neurophysiological changes. In most albinos, possibly all, there is an abnormal crossing at the chiasm with a result that the crossed fibres predominate over the uncrossed fibres. This gives rise to an abnormal visual evoked potential (VEP) (Fig. 13.4).
7 Delayed visual maturation. Some infant albinos may suffer from this condition which makes their vision appear to be worse than it actually should be (see Chapter 2).

Diagnosis
Diagnosis is based on the finding of a combination of the clinical signs, the neurophysiological changes and examination of the relatives. The tyrosinase hair bulb test detects qualitatively tyrosinase in people over 5 years old; it is not usually used clinically. Those with no evidence of tyrosinase are usually

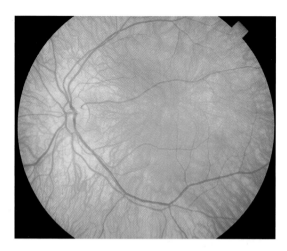

Fig. 13.1 Albinism showing hypopigmentation and macular hypoplasia.

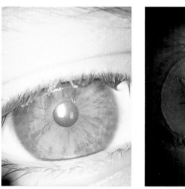

Fig. 13.2 X-linked OA in a child of Indian origin who presented with nystagmus and poor vision. This shows the brown iris with marked transillumination.

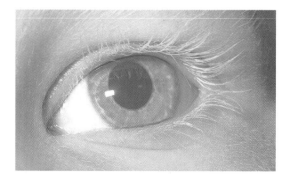

Fig. 13.3 Albinism showing white lashes and pink–blue iris.

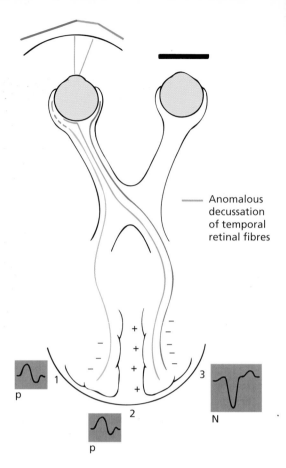

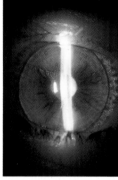

— Anomalous decussation of temporal retinal fibres

Fig. 13.4 Misrouting of the albino visual pathway. A schematic representation of the anomalous decussation of temporal retinal fibres in albinism. Most of the fibres from one eye cross at the chiasm and innervate the contralateral hemisphere. The flash VEP is recorded from three occipital electrodes (1–3), referred to a common midfrontal electrode. In albinism, flash stimulation of the left eye results in a greater activation of the right visual cortex than the left. The cortex acts as a dipole sheet and flash stimulation of the left eye gives a VEP positive peak at 80–100 ms over the left occiput (noted at P from electrode 1) and a negative peak at similar latency over the right occiput (noted at N from electrode 3). (Positive is an upward deflection.) When the right eye is stimulated the scalp distribution of positive and negative peaks is reversed. This 'crossed asymmetry' of the VEP is considered pathognomonic of albinism. In infancy, under 3 years of age, this is more clearly revealed by monocular flash stimulation, compared to pattern onset stimulation. In a normal subject a monocular flash VEP is characterized by a major midline positive peak on the midline electrode (2) at 100 ms due to the summation of more symmetrical excitation of right and left visual cortices, with smaller positive peaks over each lateral electrode.

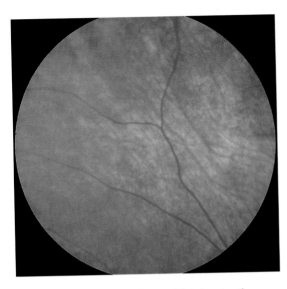

Fig. 13.5 Female carrier of X-linked OA showing the peripheral retina with mottled areas of hypopigmentation.

OCA1 albinos and are termed tyrosinase negative. Most other albinos are tyrosinase positive.

Ocular albinism

These patients are mostly X-linked recessive and the mothers may have iris transillumination defects and peripheral retinal pigment epithelial disturbances (Fig. 13.5). The ocular albinos themselves have reduced acuity, nystagmus, iris transillumination defects, foveal hypoplasia and a somewhat sparse retinal epithelium. Their skin may also be somewhat hypopigmented. Autosomal recessive cases have been described.

Oculocutaneous albinism

OCA1 are tyrosinase negative albinos with pink eyes, 'steely white' hair, and an acuity of less than 6/36. These are usually autosomal recessive.

Other albinos

There are other oculocutaneous albinos, many with more pigment in their hair, eyes and skin. Some may be autosomal dominantly inherited.

Albinism with systemic disease

1 Chediak–Higashi syndrome:

(a) partial OCA;
(b) repeated infections;
(c) autosomal recessive;
(d) bleeding diatheses;
(e) hepatosplenomegaly;
(f) neuropathies;
(g) giant cytoplasmic inclusions in leucocytes.
2 Hermansky–Pudlak syndrome:
(a) partial OCA;
(b) bleeding trait—defective platelet aggregation;
(c) pulmonary fibrosis.
3 Others:
(a) Cross syndrome;
(b) albinism and short stature.

Management of albinos

- Refraction and prescription of spectacles.
- Tinted lenses.
- Sunhat.
- Skin sun protection.
- Genetic counselling.
- Educational provision.

Congenital iris and ciliary body cysts

1 Iris stromal cysts (Fig. 13.6)
(a) anterior surface of the iris;
(b) transparent wall, vascular lining;
(c) may increase in size;
(d) may cause glaucoma;
(e) may be caused by implantation secondary to trauma.

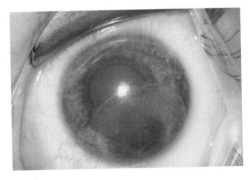

Fig. 13.6 Iris cyst. This stromal cyst recurred after local removal and eventually required a sector iridectomy.

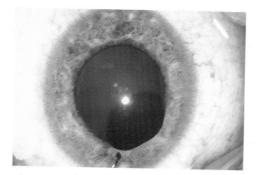

Fig. 13.7 Posterior iris cyst consisting of pigment epithelium: cysts of this type tend not to recur after simple removal with a vitrectomy machine or puncture with a yttrium–aluminium–garnet (YAG) laser.

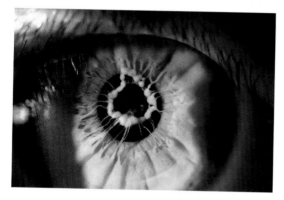

Fig. 13.8 Persistent pupillary membrane: the visual acuity was 6/12.

2 Iris pigment epithelial cyst (Fig. 13.7):
  (a) pigment lined, non-transparent;
  (b) occur at or behind the pupillary margin;
  (c) often no treatment required;
  (d) may require simple excision or puncture with yttrium–aluminium–garnet (YAG) laser.
3 Ciliary body cysts:
  (a) benign pigment cysts;
  (b) often stationary;
  (c) may require puncture or surgical removal;
  (d) cause astigmatism and amblyopia by tilting the lens.
4 Persistent pupillary membranes:
  (a) incomplete involution of the anterior, tunica vasculosa lentis;

  (b) usually collarette attachments (Fig. 13.8);
  (c) may be attached to the anterior surface of the lens;
  (d) may be associated with cataracts;
  (e) may be vascular;
  (f) may be autosomal dominant;
  (g) when mild do not impair vision;
  (h) when severe vision is impaired;
  (i) management includes refraction, prescription of spectacles or contact lenses, occlusion, pupil dilatation, surgical removal or optical iridectomy.
5 Congenital idiopathic microcoria:
  (a) small pupils that are eccentric and often drawn to one side by what appears to be a fibrous membrane (Fig. 13.9);
  (b) management
    (i) refraction if possible
    (ii) spectacles or contact lenses if necessary
    (iii) occlusion treatment
    (iv) surgical enlargement if visual potential is poor.

Aniridia

Complete aniridia
- The iris is reduced to a small stub (Fig. 13.10).
- Anterior polar cataract.
- Peripheral vascular corneal dystrophy.
- Lens dislocation.

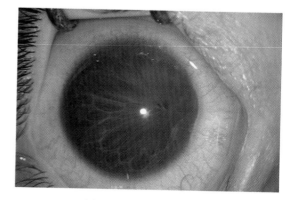

Fig. 13.9 Congenital idiopathic microcoria. The pupil in this case was so small that the eye was potentially amblyopic. The pupil was created surgically.

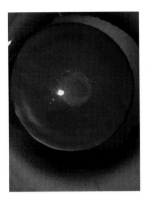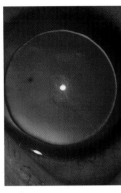

Fig. 13.10 Aniridia. No iris can be seen revealing the zonules and the lens margin. There is an anterior polar cataract in both eyes, which is most marked in the right eye.

- Glaucoma.
- Macular hypoplasia.
- Nystagmus.
- Reduced acuity usually in the region of 6/36–3/60.
- Optic nerve hypoplasia.

Partial aniridia

Similar to complete aniridia but the signs are milder and the iris is often only partly absent. Sometimes the signs are very subtle including mild iris stromal hypoplasia.

Inheritance

1 *Autosomal dominant.* This is the most common form. It is bilateral and there is variable expressivity.
2 *Autosomal recessive.* This is unusual but may occur in Gillespie's syndrome.
3 *Sporadic cases* account for about one-third of aniridics and they have in some cases been found to have deletions of 13p. These cases may be associated with Wilm's tumour, mental retardation, genitourinary abnormalities and dysmorphism (the WAGR syndrome). Sporadic patients should have detailed karyotype analysis or fluorescence *in-situ* hybridization (FISH) to look for small deletions or molecular genetic studies, otherwise all sporadic cases are followed by abdominal palpation or ultrasound studies every 3 months for up to 5 years to screen for Wilm's tumour. Wilm's tumour has been reported infrequently in familial cases.

Other associations of aniridia

- Gillespie's syndrome, anirida plus cerebellar ataxia plus mental retardation.
- Aniridia plus absent patellae.
- Others (see D. Taylor, *Paediatric Ophthalmology,* 2nd edn, 1997, Blackwell Science, Oxford; pp. 414–418).

Management

- Refraction: significant ametropia is often present.
- Prescription of glasses or occasionally contact lenses.
- Low-vision appliances.
- Educational needs.
- Protection from the sun with tinted lenses or sunhat.
- Presymptomatic detection of glaucoma.
- May require examinations under anaesthetic in infancy and early childhood.
- Most cataracts in aniridia are not functionally significant but they may become so with old age.

Box 13.1 Iris heterochromia

Congenital heterochromia
1 Ocular melanocytosis (see Chapter 6).
2 Oculodermal melanocytosis.
3 Sector iris hamartoma.
4 Congenital Horner's syndrome (ipsilateral hypopigmentation, miosis and ptosis).
5 Waardenburg's syndrome:
   (a) autosomal dominant type I — telecanthus, prominent nasal root, white forelock, deafness, locus 2q37.3;
   (b) autosomal dominant type II — same but no facial dysmorphism, locus 3p12–p14.
6 Iris sector heterochromia may be associated with Hirschsprungs's disease.
7 Iris mammillations, ectropion, naevi and freckles, see below.

Acquired heterochromia
1 Chronic uveitis.
2 Infiltration (leukaemia, other tumours).
3 Siderosis secondary to iron intraocular foreign body.
4 Haemosiderosis (long-standing hyphaema).
5 Fuchs' heterochromic cyclitis (iris lighter in colour).
6 Juvenile xanthogranuloma.

Iris ectropion

This occurs when the posterior pigment epithelium of the iris extends on to the front of the iris (Fig. 13.11).
- Congenital idiopathic.
- Secondary to glaucoma.
- Associated with congenital angle anomalies and glaucoma.
- In neurofibromatosis type 1.
- Anterior segment dysgenesis, i.e. Rieger's syndrome, etc.

Uveal tumours

1 *Iris freckles*. These are on the anterior surface of the iris with a feathery structure that does not alter iris anatomy.

2 *Iris naevi*. These are dark brown, usually homogeneous structures affecting a variable amount of the iris and they may be associated with glaucoma.

3 *Iris melanosis*:
   (a) whole iris is hyperpigmented;
   (b) smooth iris surface;
   (c) scleral pigmentation associated;
   (d) glaucoma may be associated;
   (e) some are familial.

4 *Iris mammillations*. These are villiform protuberances from the iris which are often extensive and may be associated with an iris naevus.

5 *Melanoma*. Rare in children:
   (a) iris melanomas
      (i) present early due to their visibility and hyphaema

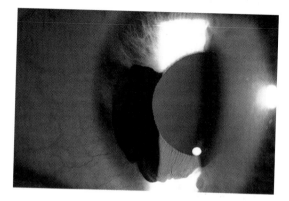

Fig. 13.11 Iris ectropion. The pupil functioned normally.

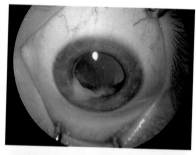

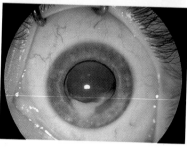

Fig. 13.12 Medulloepithelioma presenting as a felt-like structure arising in the ciliary body and involving the iris. Hyphaema may occur.

      (ii) usually relatively non-aggressive;
   (b) choroidal melanomas
      (i) usually asymptomatic
      (ii) no or slow growth
      (iii) may give rise to malignant melanomas
      (iv) malignant melanomas indicated by rapid increase in size
      (v) vascularity.

6 *Medulloepithelioma* (diktyoma) (Fig. 13.12):
   (a) unilateral;
   (b) solid;
   (c) ciliary body;
   (d) matted white appearance behind the lens;
   (e) pupil distortion;
   (f) hyphaema occasionally;
   (g) decreased vision from astigmatism;
   (h) enucleation usually necessary.

7 *Uveal haemangiomas*:
   (a) localized
      (i) usually near the optic disc
      (ii) often pigmented;
   (b) diffuse choroidal haemangiomas (tomato ketchup fundus)—Sturge–Weber's syndrome (see Chapter 24);

(c) complications
  (i) retinal detachment (serous)
  (ii) macular oedema and scarring
  (iii) treatment may be by laser, photocoagulation or radiotherapy.
8 *Choroidal osteoma*:
  (a) unilateral more frequent than bilateral;
  (b) posterior polar (Fig. 13.13);
  (c) raised;
  (d) yellow/white;
  (e) calcification shown on B scan ultrasonography;
  (f) very slow growth;
  (g) subretinal haemorrhage;
  (h) may be post-traumatic.

Uveitis

Uveitis is inflammation of the optic tract. It may be localized to certain parts of the uveal tract. Subdivisions may be defined and the conditions may be described as being acute, subacute or chronic.

Acute anterior uveitis (iritis)
Symptoms
• Pain.

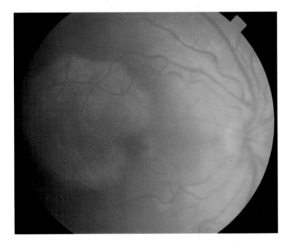

Fig. 13.13 Choroidal osteoma probably of traumatic origin. This unilateral lesion presented because of poor vision found at a routine school test. There was also a posterior subcapsular cataract. The fundus lesion had high echogenicity on ultrasound studies.

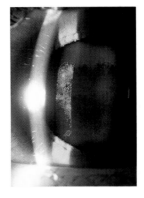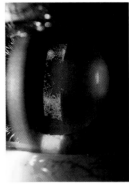

Fig. 13.14 Acute anterior uveitis with fibrinous exudate on the anterior surface of the lens.

• Redness.
• Photophobia.

Signs
• Anterior chamber flare and cells.
• Keratic precipitates (KP) (Fig. 13.14).
• Vision reduction due to macular oedema, glaucoma, anterior chamber turbidity, iridocyclitis.
• Iridocyclitis can be seen from cells behind the lens.

Causes of acute anterior uveitis
• Trauma.
• Infectious diseases:
  (a) exanthemata;
  (b) brucellosis;
  (c) cat scratch disease;
  (d) herpes simplex;
  (e) infectious mononucleosis;
  (f) Kawasaki's disease (mucocutaneous lymph node syndrome) — a systemic vasculitis affecting children which presents with
    (i) a fever
    (ii) stomatitis
    (iii) palmar erythema
    (iv) lymphadenopathy
    (v) myocarditis
    (vi) bilateral conjunctivitis
    (vii) uveitis;
  (g) Lyme disease;
  (h) spondyloarthropathies;

(i) ankylosing spondylitis;

(j) psoriatic arthritis;

(k) inflammatory bowel disease (Crohn's and ulcerative colitis);

(l) Reiter's syndrome;

(m) Behçet's disease.

Chronic anterior uveitis

Causes

- Trauma.
- Leprosy.
- Onchocerciasis.
- Juvenile rheumatoid arthritis (Still's disease):
  (a) the most common cause in childhood;
  (b) onset before 16 years of age;
  (c) pauciarticular—four joints or less in the first 3 months;
  (d) polyarticular—five or more joints in the first 3 months;
  (e) acute febrile—with a systemic illness.

Iridocyclitis in juvenile rheumatoid arthritis

- Most frequent in pauciarticular juvenile rheumatoid arthritis with rheumatoid factor negative and positive antinuclear antibody and negative human leucocyte antigen (HLA)-B27.
- Females more frequently affected than males.
- Early onset, before 10 years.

Box 13.2 The Still's disease tetrad

1 Chronic mild, often asymptomatic uveitis.
2 Band keratopathy (Fig. 13.15).
3 Cataract.
4 Glaucoma.

Complications such as posterior synechiae and associated cataract formation together with glaucoma may be preventable by early presymptomatic treatment. Therefore, it is appropriate to screen Still's patients at risk.

- Systemic onset—annually.
- Polyarticular forms 6-monthly.
- Pauciarticular forms 3-monthly.
- Pauciarticular forms who are antinuclear antibody (ANA) positive every 2 months until 7 years

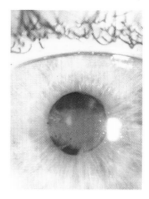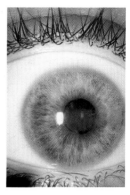

Fig. 13.15 Still's disease. This patient presented because the parents noticed a white spot on the cornea, which was due to the band keratopathy associated with chronic uveitis with posterior synechiae. She had the pauciarticular form of Still's disease and later developed cataracts.

after the onset of the condition. Some patients who are obviously in remission early may forego the screening earlier.

Management of anterior uveitis

1 Mydriatics. It is best to treat with short-acting mydriatics so that the pupil moves. Patients without posterior synechiae but who are at high risk may be best treated with very short-acting mydriatics given at night so that the effects of the associated cycloplegia do not trouble them unnecessarily.

2 Topical cortical steroids by drops, when cells are present in the anterior chamber. For chronic flare alone treatment is not usually successful. For acute exacerbations the steroids may need to be given every hour with frequent ophthalmological checks.

3 For acute exacerbations subtenons injections of depo steroids or soluble steroids or a short course of systemic steroids, starting with a high dose and reducing quite quickly, may be appropriate. Systemic immunosuppressive treatment may be helpful in severe chronic cases.

4 Band keratopathy may require excimer laser ablation, corneal scraping or the use of ethylenediaminetetraacetic acid (EDTA) chelating agent.

5 Cataract surgery in chronic anterior uveitis. Cataract surgery can be complicated by severe postoperative uveitis with vitreous organisation. In

most cases of severe uveitis a lensectomy/vitrectomy approach is indicated. Only very mild cases may be treated with lens aspiration with preservation of the posterior capsule. In all cases it is appropriate to do one or two large peripheral iridectomies or a broad iridectomy, and all cases should be covered by intensive topical and systemic steroids around the time of surgery.

6 Glaucoma may be treated by:
    (a) iridectomy if there is pupil block;
    (b) topical antihypertensive agents;
    (c) acetazolamide;
    (d) trabeculodialysis;
    (e) trabeculectomy enhanced with antimitotic agents or a drainage tube procedure.

7 Macula oedema is treated by improved control of the uveitis and, in some cases, by non-steroidal anti-inflammatory agents.

Prognosis

In all patients the prognosis should be very guarded from the beginning. At least 25% of patients with chronic uveitis associated with juvenile rheumatoid arthritis have a poor visual prognosis.

Sarcoidosis

• Granulomatous uveitis (Fig. 13.16) with large 'mutton fat' KP.
• Arthropathy.
• Skin rash.
• Hepatosplenomegaly.

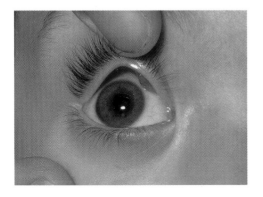

Fig. 13.16 Sarcoidosis showing a very large KP just below the pupils. There are posterior synechiae and the iris is engorged.

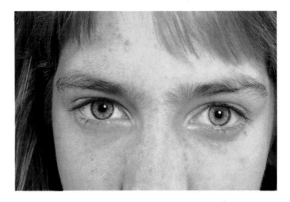

Fig. 13.17 Fuchs' heterochromic iridocyclitis. This girl presented because of mildly blurred vision in the left eye and heterochromia, which her parents had noticed. She had a mild chronic anterior uveitis without synechiae: a cataract developed.

Diagnosis is suggested by finding a negative Mantoux test, a raised serum angiotensin-converting enzyme or a positive Kweim test. The treatment of the uveitis is similar to the treatment of the iritis associated with juvenile rheumatoid arthritis with a greater use of systemic steroids and only rarely is chemotherapy indicated.

Fuchs' heterochromic cyclitis

• A chronic anterior uveitis with iris hypopigmentation.
• Unusual in childhood.
• Slow painless loss of vision.
• Heterochromia (Fig. 13.17).
• Unilateral, usually.
• Cataract.
• Fine KPs.
• White eye.
• Iris transillumination defects.
• May be associated with morphoea.
• Glaucoma frequent and refractory to topical therapy.

Tuberculosis

• Anterior granulomatous uveitis with retinochoroiditis.
• Subacute endophthalmitis.
• Usually evidence of systemic tuberculosis.

Syphilis

Although rare in childhood, it should be suspected in the appropriate social situation, especially when there is an associated interstitial keratitis.

Pars planitis (intermediate uveitis)

This is a condition in which there is a chronic uveitis affecting the ciliary body and vitreous, and the pars plana.

- Usually in teenagers.
- Bilateral/asymmetrical.
- Symptoms of floaters or reduced vision if cystoid macular oedema develops.
- Redness, pain and photophobia rare.
- Examination shows white deposits in the peripheral parts of the anterior vitreous.
- Minimal flare or cells.
- Posterior synechiae sometimes.
- Associated retinal vasculitis.

Complications

- Cystoid macular oedema.
- Cataract secondary to glaucoma.
- Optic disc neovascularisation.
- Vitreous haemorrhage.
- Retinal detachment.

Cause

Unknown.

Treatment

If asymptomatic and vision excellent, no treatment necessary. If acuity is reduced, subtenons or systemic steroids may be helpful.

Posterior uveitis

Toxocara

- Endophthalmitis.
- Retinal granuloma (Fig. 13.18)
- Caused by *Toxocara canis* larvae.
- Always unilateral.
- Males more frequent than females.

Presenting symptoms

- Strabismus.
- Leucocoria.
- Failed school screening examination.

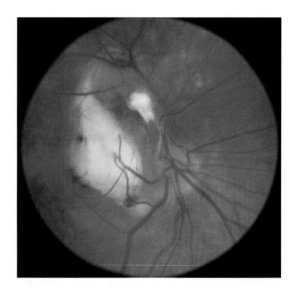

Fig. 13.18 *Toxocara*. This 5-year-old child failed his school eye test and was found to have a raised peripapillary lesion between the optic disc and the macula in his left eye. At this stage there was minimal active inflammation.

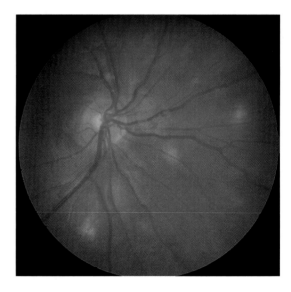

Fig. 13.19 Miliary tuberculosis with focal choroidal lesion.

Signs

- Marked vitreous haze.
- Retinal choroidal granuloma.
- Retinal detachment.

Diagnosis

The main differential diagnosis is with retinoblastoma.

• Enzyme-linked immunosorbent assay (ELISA) *Toxocara* test. It must be remembered that a large proportion of older children have positive anti-*Toxocara* antibodies.

• Retinoblastoma can often be differentiated by finding calcium on computerized tomography scanning, which is infrequent in *Toxocara*.

Treatment

Treatment rarely makes any difference to this condition. Steroids may suppress the inflammation but antihelminthics do not help. Enucleation should only be performed when the diagnosis of retinoblastoma cannot be excluded and the eye is blind and painful.

Endophthalmitis, infective causes and toxoplasmosis (see Chapter 5)

Sympathetic ophthalmia

Sympathetic ophthalmia is usually related to trauma, most often severe penetrating trauma involving damage to the uvea. It is now rare in this situation and also occurs very rarely following intraocular surgery. The symptoms are of pain, photophobia, a decrease in vision, worsening inflammation of the traumatised eye and bilateral iritis with viscous exudate. Systemic effects may occur such as poliosis (white lashes) and vitilligo. Treatment is usually unrewarding.

Sarcoidosis

Posterior uveitis is unusual in sarcoidosis but there may be a form of retinal vasculitis with periphlebitis characterized by venous sheathing and chorioretinal nodules, vitreous cells, occasional vitreous haemorrhage and neovascularisation. Optic nerve involvement has been described.

Choroidal tuberculosis

With miliary tuberculosis, multiple choroidal white spots may occur (Fig. 13.19).

14: Lens

Anatomy and embryology

The crystalline lens is a biconvex refracting structure that lies posterior to the iris and anterior to the vitreous humour, suspended by zonules extending from the ciliary body. At birth the lens has an equatorial diameter of 6.5 mm and anterior–posterior depth of 3.5 mm. By adulthood the equatorial diameter is 9 mm and the anterior–posterior depth 5 mm. The posterior surface of the lens vesicle is lined by columnar epithelial cells which give rise to the primary lens fibres. The lens capsule is formed from the deposition of basement membrane material of the lens epithelium.

Developmental anomalies

A wide range of developmental defects give rise to anomalies of the lens size, shape, position and optical clarity. These include the following.
• *Congenital aphakia.* This may come about either by primary failure of lens development or secondary to spontaneous lens absorption. In either case, visual acuity is usually poor due to maldevelopment of other structures of the eye.
• *Duplication of the lens* is a rare anomaly that may be associated with metaplasia of the cornea and colobomas.
• *Lens colobomas* may occur as an isolated anomaly (usually unilateral) or in association with other colobomatous defects (usually bilateral) (Fig. 14.1).
• *Microspherophakia* (Fig. 14.2) is an anomaly in which the lens is reduced in diameter and spherical in shape. It may occur as an isolated anomaly or as part of the Weill–Marchesani syndrome.
• *Lenticonus* is an axial deformity of the posterior lens surface that may be associated with a developmental cataract. It is usually unilateral and may be inherited as an autosomal recessive or X-linked

recessive trait.
• *Anterior lenticonus* is an axial deformity of the anterior capsule that usually does not evolve into a visually significant cataract but may be associated with Alport's syndrome. Alport's syndrome — hereditary nephritis with sensorineural deafness — is inherited as an X-linked trait and is due to a mutation in the *COL4A5* collagen gene at Xq22.
• *Remnants of the tunica vasculosa lentis.* These may be seen as a dot on the posterior surface of the lens or as an extensive network of vascular remnants adherent to the posterior lens capsules (especially in the premature infant).

Persistent hyperplastic primary vitreous (PHPV) (see Chapter 16)

This term is used to describe a wide spectrum of congenital anomalies that include the following:
• microphthalmos;
• shallow anterior chamber;
• elongated ciliary processes;
• cataract;
• retinal detachment;
• retrolental plaque;
• intralenticular haemorrhage.

This is usually a unilateral condition and the cataract may be visually insignificant at birth but progressive. Good visual acuity results may be obtained in some cases but the postoperative complication rate is high. Glaucoma occurs frequently (Fig. 14.3).

Dislocated lenses

Luxation refers to complete dislocation from its normal pupillary position. Subluxation represents only a partial displacement. In children, subluxation may result in reduced visual acuity and secondary

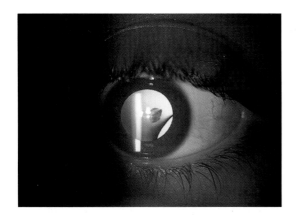

Fig. 14.1 Lens coloboma.

The features of homocystinuria (Fig. 14.4) are:
- arachnodactyly;
- malar flush;
- fair hair;
- mental retardation;
- thromboembolic events;
- ectopia lentis (usually dislocating inferiorly and/ or anteriorly.

Because affected patients are normal at birth, early diagnosis and treatment are essential. Treatment of these patients is with:
- high doses of pyridoxine;
- betaine;

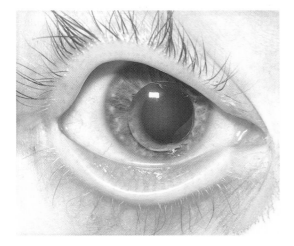

Fig. 14.2 Microspherophakia with anterior dislocation.

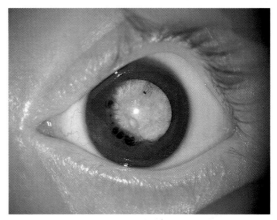

Fig. 14.3 Marked vascular PHPV with multiple vessels between the fibrous plaque, the lens and the iris.

amblyopia. Luxation of the lens anteriorly may be associated with pupil-block glaucoma or corneal oedema. Causes of dislocated lenses include the following.

Homocystinuria

This is a disease of methionine metabolism due to deficiency of cystathionine-B-synthetase. Affected patients have elevated levels of homocystine and methionine in blood and urine. The diagnosis may be established with a urine sodium nitroprusside test or by measuring homocystine in the urine following methionine loading.

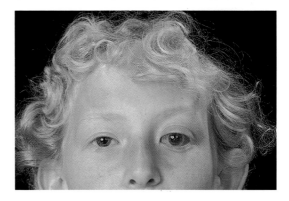

Fig. 14.4 Homocystinuria. A fair-haired boy with chronic glaucoma following unreported anterior dislocation of the lens.

• low methionine;
• high-cysteine diet.

They must be kept well hydrated during surgery. Any surgery carries a risk of thromboembolic episodes.

Marfan's syndrome

Marfan's syndrome is the most common cause of ectopia lentis in childhood. It is inherited as an autosomal dominant disorder as a result of mutation of the fibrillin gene on chromosome 15q21.1. Its clinical features include the following.

• *Cardiac*—dilatation of the aortic route, microvalve prolapse, aortic aneurysm.

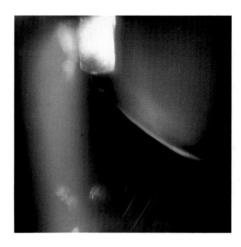

Fig. 14.6 Marfan's syndrome. Dislocated lens with intact stretched zonule.

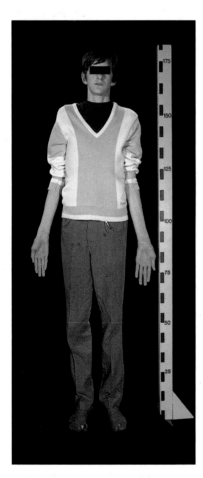

Fig. 14.5 Marfan's syndrome. At the age of 15 years he is 1.75 m tall. He has very long limbs, arachnodactyly and pectus excavatum.

• *Skeletal*—excessive height, arachnodactyly, scoliosis and chest wall deformities (Fig. 14.5).
• *Ocular*—ectopia lentis (usually dislocating superiorly), cataract, high myopia, retinal detachment. The high myopia seen in Marfan's syndrome is not always lenticular but may be axial. Axial myopia predisposes the patient to a high risk of retinal detachment with or without cataract surgery (Fig. 14.6).

Weill–Marchesani syndrome

The *Weill–Marchesani syndrome* is a rare disorder inherited as an autosomal recessive trait, although autosomal dominant inheritance has also been found. Its clinical features are:

• short stature;
• brachycephaly;
• stubby fingers and toes;
• spherophakia (dislocation is usually anterior);
• lenticular myopia.

Other syndromes in which ectopia lentis may occur include the following:

• aniridia;
• ectopia lentis et pupillae — autosomal recessive syndrome with lens and pupil displacement in the opposite direction;
• simple ectopia lentis — inherited as an isolated autosomal dominant trait;

- sulphite oxidase deficiency—associated with dislocated lenses, progressive muscular rigidity and early death;
- trauma;
- glaucoma;
- xanthine oxidase deficiency—associated with low levels of serum uric acid.

Treatment of dislocated lenses

Treatment of dislocated lenses is necessary to ensure good visual acuity and to prevent amblyopia. In addition, surgical removal of the lens may be necessary when the dislocation is anterior in order to prevent damage to the cornea and to prevent glaucoma.

Surgical complications have been reduced by the introduction of closed-eye lensectomy–vitrectomy techniques. Treatment may include the following.
- *Spectacle correction*—this may be limited by high refractive errors that make the spectacles difficult for the child to wear.
- *Contact lenses*—these are particularly useful in the treatment of the high myope or aphake.
- *Dilatation of the pupil* — may be used both for optical purposes as well as repositioning an anterior displaced lens.
- *Surgery* — lensectomy–vitrectomy techniques utilising a limbal or pars plana approach. Retinal detachment is the most significant risk associated with this surgery.
- *Yttrium–aluminium–garnet (YAG) laser lysis of the lens zonules* — may be used to relocate the lens bisecting the pupil.

Cataracts

Any opacity of the crystalline lens is referred to as a cataract. Because of the association of form deprivation amblyopia with cataracts in early infancy, these represent an important treatable cause of visual disability in children. Early diagnosis and treatment is essential if irreparable visual loss is to be prevented.

Aetiology

In many cases no aetiology for the cataract may be determined. However, careful inspection of the morphology of the cataract, examination of the parents and appropriate laboratory investigations may establish a diagnosis in many patients.

Common causes of cataracts in children include:
- inherited;
- autosomal recessive inheritance — uncommon except in metabolic disorder;
- autosomal dominant—anterior polar, lamellar—may be associated with microphthalmos;
- X-linked recessive — Lowe's syndrome, Nance–Horan syndrome, Lenz syndrome.

Intrauterine infections

Mandatory immunization programmes have significantly reduced the prevalence rate of the rubella embryopathy syndrome. Nevertheless, the child with dense unilateral or bilateral cataracts should be investigated for the possibility of a rubella infection. This may be tested with rubella immunoglobulin G (IgG) and IgM antibodies measured in both the mother and the child.

Metabolic disorders

A wide variety of metabolic disorders are associated with cataract formation. These include the following.
- *Galactosaemia*—this is caused by a mutation of the gene on the short arm of chromosome 9 coding for galactose-1-phosphate uridyl-transferase. These patients may present with diarrhoea, vomiting, jaundice, hepatomegaly and Gram-positive septicaemia. Cataracts are not usually detected until the child is systemically unwell. Heterozygotes for galactosaemia may be at increased risk for cataract formation in early adulthood.

Galactose-restricted diets may prevent cataract formation when instituted early in the course of the disease (Fig. 14.7).
- *Wilson's disease* — a disorder of iron metabolism associated with subcapsular sunflower cataracts (Fig. 14.8).
- *Hypocalcaemia* — associated with seizures, failure to thrive and fine white punctate lens opacities (Fig. 14.9).
- *Diabetes mellitus* — children with juvenile diabetes frequently present as teenagers with cortical opacities.

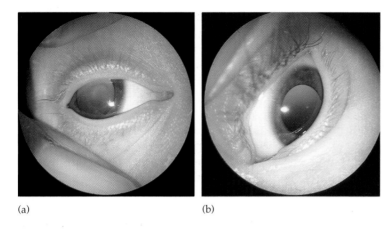

(a)   (b)

Fig. 14.7 (a) 'Oil-droplet cataract' in galactosaemia is a central refractive change in the lens. (b) After early dietary treatment the 'cataract' had disappeared (same patient).

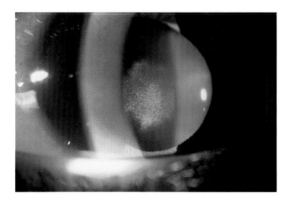

Fig. 14.8 Wilson's disease—'sunflower' cataract.

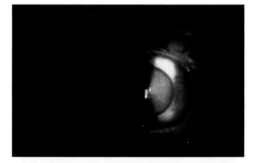

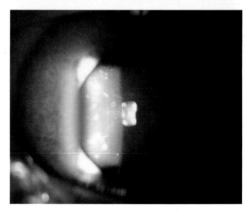

Fig. 14.9 Hypocalcaemic cataract—punctate dots.

- *Hypoglycaemia* — in the early infant period may result in lens opacities that are reversible.
- *Autosomal recessive syndrome* with exercise-related lactic acidosis, mitochondrial cytopathy and hypertrophic cardiomyopathy and congenital cataract.

Chromosome abnormalities and other syndromes

- *Trisomy 21*—mature cataracts frequent in infancy.
- *Cri du chat*—caused by the partial deletion of the short arm of chromosome 5 associated with microcephaly, low-set ears and cardiac malformations.
- *Hallermann–Streiff–François syndrome*—associated with dyscephaly, short stature, hypotrichosis, dental anomalies, blue sclera and congenital cataract (Fig. 14.10).

- *Martsolf syndrome* — mental retardation, micrognathia, brachycephaly, flat maxilla, broad sternum and talipes.
- *The Marinesco–Sjögren syndrome*—mental retardation, cerebellar ataxia, myopathy.

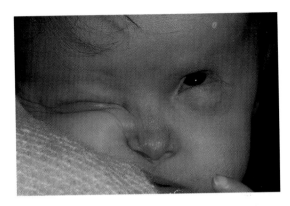

Fig. 14.10 Hallermann–Streiff–François syndrome showing a small nose with prominent veins. Baldness and progeria are common.

- *Chondrodysplasia punctata* — seen in three forms: autosomal recessive, X-linked dominant and autosomal dominant.
- *X-linked cataract*, spasticity and mental retardation.
- *Autosomal recessive cerebro-oculo-facio-skeletal syndrome* — mental retardation, microcephaly, joint contractions, micrognathia, sloping forehead and cataract.
- *Czeizel–Lowry syndrome* — microcephaly, Perthes' disease of the hip and cataract.
- *Killian–Pallister–Mosaic syndrome* — coarse facial features, hypertelorism, saggy cheeks, sparse hair and cataract. Tetrasomy of the short arm of chromosome 12.
- *Progressive spinocerebellar ataxia*, deafness, peripheral neuropathy and cataract.
- *Proximal myopathy* with facial, ocular and bulbar weakness, hypogonadism, ataxia and cataract.
- *Pollitt syndrome* — mental retardation, short stature, scaly skin and cataract.
- *Schwarz–Jampel syndrome* — congenital myotonic myopathy, ptosis, skeletal defects, microphthalmos and cataract.
- *Cataract*, mental retardation, microdontia, pectus excavation and hypertrichosis.
- *Velo-cardio-facial syndrome* — prominent nose, notched alae nasae, micrognathia and cleft palate.
- *Others*—see D. Taylor (ed.), *Paediatric Ophthalmology*, 2nd edn, 1997, Blackwell Science, Oxford.

Steroid and radiation cataract

Chronic corticosteroid therapy may produce posterior subcapsular cataracts that may regress if steroid therapy is promptly discontinued. Similar cataracts may develop in children treated with radiation therapy to the orbital region (Fig. 14.11).

Uveitis

Posterior subcapsular cataracts commonly develop in association with juvenile rheumatoid arthritis and pars planitis.

Prematurity

Transient opacities along the posterior lens suture have been reported in premature infants.

Treatment

Pre-operative evaluation

In the case of binocular congenital or early developmental cataracts early surgery is clearly indicated when the opacities completely occlude the visual axis. In the case of partial cataracts it is sometimes a more difficult decision to determine if the cataracts are significantly amblyogenic. The morphology of the cataract may be helpful: nuclear cataracts are more amblyogenic than lamellar (Figs 14.12 & 14.13). Nevertheless, repeated re-evaluation of the patient may be necessary in determining whether the patient with partial cataracts requires surgery.

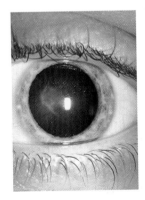
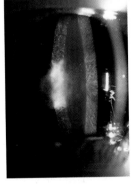

Fig. 14.11 Posterior subcapsular cataract in a child with treated leukaemia. This may be due to steroid treatment, chemotherapy or radiotherapy.

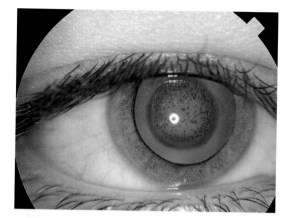

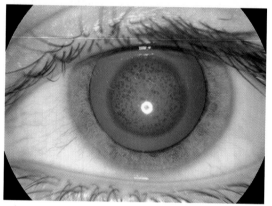

Fig. 14.12 Bilateral symmetrical lamellar cataracts in retroillumination. The acuity is 6/9 in both eyes.

Assessment of the other structures of the eye are important to determine if associated anomalies may preclude a good visual result.

Monocular congenital cataracts

Whether or not monocular congenital cataracts should be routinely surgically removed remains controversial. Although some patients operated on in the first few months of life have been rehabilitated with excellent visual acuities, most patients with monocular congenital cataracts continue to exhibit poor visual acuity. The parents need to be advised of the difficulty in obtaining long-term good visual results.

Systemic evaluation

Systemic evaluation of the patient with congenital or developmental cataracts should be co-ordinated with a paediatrician. In some cases the morphology of the lens opacity (e.g. in the case of PHPV) will clearly indicate that no systemic evaluation is necessary. In other cases evaluation for metabolic or infectious causes is indicated.

Surgery

For infants, the surgical removal of monocular or binocular congenital cataracts by closed-eye lensectomy–vitrectomy techniques are most appropriate (Fig. 14.14). These provide for a clear visual axis that

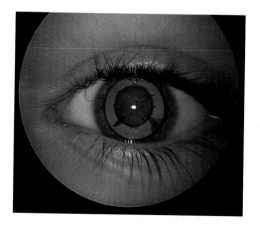

Fig. 14.13 Lamellar cataract with riders; the acuity is 6/24.

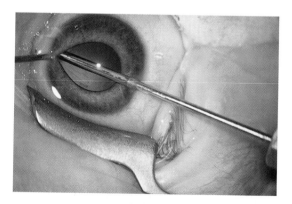

Fig. 14.14 Lensectomy showing the iris retracted by an irrigating cystitome and the vitrectomy machine removing the cortex and capsule underneath this area. Using a two-handed technique may help to get a fuller clearance of the lens and capsule.

permits routine retinoscopy in the postoperative period. This technique has not been associated with a significant incidence of retinal detachment, although longer follow-up studies are necessary.

In the older child (more than 2 years of age), where implantation of an intraocular lens may be considered, standard lens aspiration techniques may be preferred.

YAG laser capsulotomy may be necessary in a high percentage of these patients in the immediate postoperative period due to posterior capsule opacification (Figs 14.15 & 14.16).

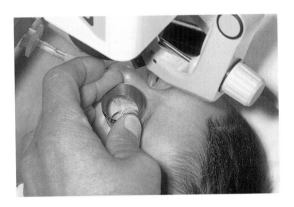

Fig. 14.15 Horizontally mounted YAG laser. Using a contact lens (in this case a gonioscopy lens) patients can be treated easily under general anaesthetic.

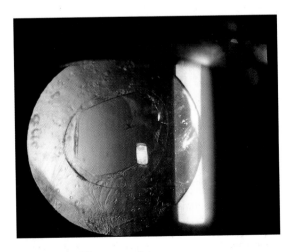

Fig. 14.16 YAG laser capsulotomy.

Phakoemulsification techniques are rarely indicated in children.

Aphakic correction

Precise correction of the refractive error resulting from paediatric aphakia is necessary if good visual acuity results are to be obtained. Periodic changes in the contact lenses will be necessary as eye growth occurs and the refractive error decreases. The aphakic may be corrected by the following.

Spectacles

Primarily used in bilateral aphakia but occasionally in the contact lens intolerant monocular aphake. One advantage of spectacles is their relative low cost. Disadvantages include the difficulty of fitting a heavy spectacle on a young infant whose small nose will not support many spectacle frames.

Contact lenses

In most cases contact lenses remain the standard method for optical correction of both monocular and binocular aphakia in infancy. Soft, gas permeable and even hard lenses have been utilized in these patients. Silicone lenses have been especially efficacious in the first few months of life. Frequent lens loss and the need to change lens power as the result of eye growth makes this a costly procedure. Although keratitis and corneal scarring have been reported in the paediatric aphakic patient it is surprising how infrequent these problems are clinically significant (Fig. 14.17).

Epikeratophakia

This procedure, using a lamellar on-lay corneal graft, has proved disappointing. It is rarely utilised at the present time.

Intraocular lenses

Intraocular lenses are being used increasingly in the treatment of the child with developmental or traumatic rather than congenital cataracts. Many authorities believe they are appropriate even in the child as young as the age of 2 years. At this age most of the eye growth is complete and the prediction of lens power that will be necessary for a child as an adult is less problematical. The use of

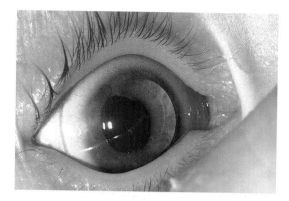

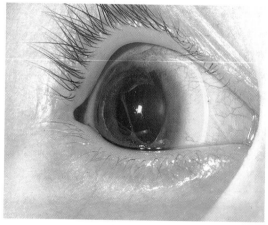

Fig. 14.17 Aphakic contact lenses are the treatment of choice in infant aphakia (see text).

intraocular lenses in congenital cataracts remains controversial.

Primary implantation at the time of initial surgery in the first few weeks of life seems unwise. Obviously the question of what power of intraocular lens to use in these children is complicated by the normal ocular growth pattern, the microphthalmos seen in many of these patients and the question of whether the intraocular lens itself alters the normal growth pattern.

Thus, in most cases, true congenital cataracts are not treated with primary intraocular lens implantation, although secondary lens procedures are becoming more popular for the older child with good vision.

In the case of the older child with traumatic cataracts, intraocular lenses are being used as the standard treatment for aphakia. Currently, an 'in-the-bag' single piece PMMA lens is most commonly used (Fig. 14.18).

Amblyopia treatment

The greatest obstacle to obtaining good visual acuity in the patient with monocular or binocular congenital cataracts is form-deprivation amblyopia. In order to obtain good visual acuity results, surgery must be completed in the first few months of life and the visual axis kept clear postoperatively. Periodic re-evaluation of the refractive error with refitting of the appropriate contact lens is mandatory.

Even so, a significant percentage of monocular congenital cataracts treated in this manner will not develop good visual acuity. Binocular cases will generally do better, but many will never obtain normal visual acuity levels.

Monocular form deprivation

Most studies suggest that surgery must be completed in the first 2–3 months of life if good visual acuity is to be obtained. Immediate optical correction and patching therapy needs to be instituted in the postoperative period. Part-time patching

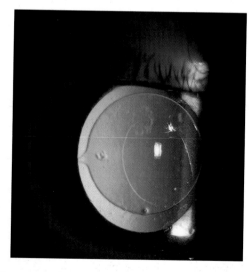

Fig. 14.18 Intraocular lens. This one-piece PMMA lens is placed in-the-bag through a capsulorhexis. YAG laser treatment is usually required within a few weeks of surgery.

(50–70% of waking hours) is usually utilized in order to avoid the risk of occlusion amblyopia in the fixing eye (rare) and, more importantly, the induction of nystagmus in the fixing eye (Fig. 14.19).

Binocular form deprivation

If surgery and visual rehabilitation of the binocular congenital cataract patient is completed before nystagmus appears, often little or no significant binocular form-deprivation amblyopia will be apparent. Once nystagmus supervenes, however, visual acuity levels are significantly reduced even with aggressive therapy. In many cases of binocular form deprivation, monocular deprivation is also seen and patching of the preferred fixing eye needs to be undertaken if visual acuity results are to be equalised. Complications of cataract surgery in children are significant and not always comparable to those seen in adults. These complications include the following.

• *Amblyopia.* As already discussed, amblyopia is the major obstacle to obtaining good visual acuity in both monocular and binocular congenital cataracts. This comes about due to the occlusion of the visual axis caused by the cataract. Additionally, anisometropia and strabismus may add additional amblyogenic factors.

• *Capsular opacification.* Opacification of the posterior capsule in the infant eye occurs in nearly 100%

of cases within the first few weeks or months postoperatively. It is for this reason that lensectomy–vitrectomy techniques were introduced to provide a means of posterior capsulectomy at the time of surgery.

If lens aspiration techniques are utilized, YAG posterior capsulectomies will be frequently required in the postoperative period.

• *Corneal oedema.* Some degree of corneal oedema is commonly seen immediately following cataract surgery in children, particularly if an intrastromal infusion cannula is utilized. In most cases it spontaneously resolves and is not a long-lasting complication.

• *Cystoid macular oedema.* Rarely reported in children.

• *Endophthalmitis.* Although uncommon, endophthalmitis does occur in the paediatric cataract patient. A concurrent nasolacrimal duct obstruction, upper respiratory infection or periorbital skin disorder may predispose to the complication. Visual results are usually poor in these patients (Fig. 14.20).

• *Glaucoma.* This remains a major complication in the paediatric aphakic patient. Its prevalence rate may be as high as 20–30% in congenital cataract patients. An increased risk is associated with microphthalmos, PHPV and nuclear cataracts. It may not be apparent until several years following surgery. Routine measurement of intraocular

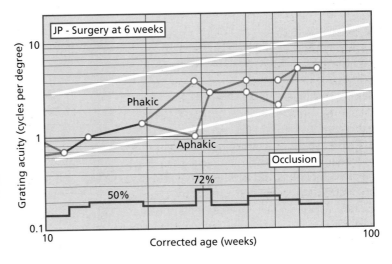

Fig. 14.19 Monocular cataract occlusion regimen. The acuities of the phakic (blue) and aphakic (pink) eye have been monitored using Keeler cards. Initially the acuities in the two eyes were the same and the child was maintained on a 50% of waking hours occlusion regimen. When the aphakic eye fell behind the phakic eye, the amount of occlusion (bottom line) was increased to a maximum of 72% in this case.

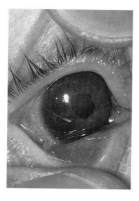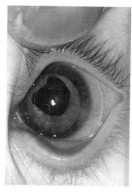

Fig. 14.20 Endophthalmitis of the right eye. This child had bilateral cataracts and microcoria. The left eye had been operated successfully and a larger pupil created. The right developed endophthalmitis from the first postoperative day.

pressure, examination of the optic disc and re-evaluation of the refractive error is recommended to detect glaucoma as early as possible. A rapid decrease in the hyperopic prescription in an aphakic eye should suggest a possibility of associated glaucoma. The treatment of glaucoma associated with paediatric aphakia remains disappointing.

• *Irregular pupils.* Some irregularity of the pupil is common following cataract surgery in children but is rarely visually significant. Occasionally in the treatment of PHPV a section of iris will have to be resected during removal of the stiff membranous tissue, applying traction to the ciliary processes (Fig. 14.21).

• *Nystagmus.* Bilateral nystagmus occurs in a significant proportion of children with binocular congenital cataracts. It suggests the presence of binocular form-deprivation amblyopia. Nystagmus may also occur in the monocular congenital cataract patient. It may be either monocular or binocular, and in either case carries a poor prognosis.

• *Retinal detachment.* Since the introduction of lensectomy–vitrectomy techniques two decades ago the prevalence of retinal detachments has remained low in paediatric aphakic patients. It should be recalled, however, that previous studies of retinal detachment following other surgical techniques for lens removal emphasized that detachment may not occur until the third and even fourth decade following surgery. Long-term studies are necessary before it can be concluded that retinal detachment is not a significant risk in the patient who undergoes lensectomy–vitrectomy in the treatment of congenital cataract.

• *Strabismus.* Strabismus (usually esotropia) is often the presenting sign in a child with monocular congenital cataract. It may also occur following surgical removal of the lens. Although rarely seen preoperatively in the binocular congenital cataract case it may occur during the course of postoperative treatment. Strabismus adds one more amblyogenic factor to the problem of visual rehabilitation in these patients.

Visual results

In the last two decades visual results in congenital and developmental cataracts have been remarkably improved. This is due to a combination of factors including emphasis on early detection of cataracts, improved surgical techniques for removal, better and more available aphakic contact lenses and the use of intraocular lenses in select cases. In the case of congenital cataracts, the single most important factor determining the visual outcome is early detection, which emphasises the need for specific examination of all newborn infants with a direct ophthalmoscope or retinoscope to assess the presence or absence of lens opacities as soon as possible. The results in binocular congenital cataracts are

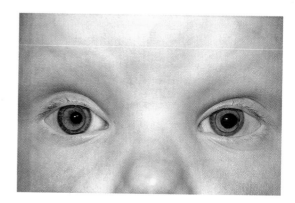

Fig. 14.21 Irregular pupil in the left eye secondary to iris damage during surgery.

now usually quite good and although legal blindness or serious visual impairment has been bilateral reduced congenital cataract 0remains a significant problem.

Results in the treatment of monocular congenital cataract patients are less good but promising. The most significant postoperative complication that threatens to abolish an initially good visual acuity result is glaucoma.

15: Glaucoma

Glaucoma in childhood is relatively infrequent. Paediatric glaucoma represents a complex collection of diverse pathophysiological entities. Most forms of paediatric glaucoma are the result of structural maldevelopment of the anterior segment and angle structures. Regardless of the pathophysiological mechanism, most paediatric glaucomas share similar signs and symptoms, many of which differ markedly from adult glaucoma.

Enlargement of the globe

Infant sclera and cornea are much less rigid, more elastic and distensible than in adults. High intraocular pressure may produce distention, enlargement and thinning of the outer walls of the eye. This change rarely occurs in glaucomas beginning after the age of 2 years (Fig. 15.1)

Corneal changes

Corneal enlargement is tolerated by the epithelium and stroma initially but not by the endothelium and Descemet's membrane. As stretching of the cornea progresses, breaks in Descemet's membrane occur (Haab's striae). They may be circumferential or linear. As the result of these breaks corneal oedema may occur. Most of the symptoms of infantile glaucomas are the result of this oedematous process (Fig. 15.2).

Photophobia/tearing

As opacification and enlargement of the cornea occurs photophobia is likely to accompany it. Tearing can be marked and may in some circumstances be misdiagnosed as obstruction of the nasolacrimal drainage system.

Optic disc cupping

Optic disc cupping occurs in infantile glaucomas just as it does in the older patient. However, cupping may be reversible in the young patient; thus, the degree to which the optic nerve is cupped is not always a good prognostic indicator.

Refractive changes and strabismus

Stretching of the cornea and sclera may lead to significant refractive errors. Correcting these is important if amblyopia is to be avoided. Strabismus may occur, especially when glaucoma is asymmetrical and this too may lead to amblyopia. A sudden myopic shift in the young aphake should suggest the possibility of glaucoma.

Classification

No single classification of paediatric glaucomas is available. In most classifications, however, the glaucomas are divided into primary and secondary disorders. In primary glaucomas the elevation in intraocular pressure comes about as the result of an intrinsic disorder of aqueous outflow. In contrast, in secondary glaucomas the glaucoma is associated with a disease process that may involve other regions of the eye and body. This chapter utilises an anatomical classification based on that proposed by D. Hoskins.

Primary congenital glaucoma (trabeculodysgenesis: primary infantile glaucoma)

This is the most common form of glaucoma in children, occurring in one in 10 000 births. The disease is usually bilateral but may be asymmetrical or even unilateral. In the USA and the UK it is more

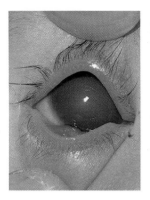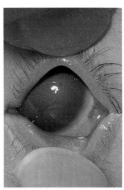

Fig. 15.1 Bilateral severe buphthalmos in a neonate with enlarged 'steamy' corneas.

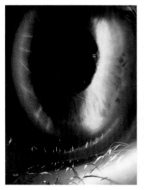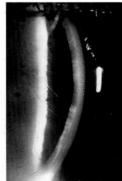

Fig. 15.2 Splits in Descemet's membrane have corneal oedema at their edges for many months giving rise to linear opacities (Haab's striae) which are present even when the intraocular pressure is controlled.

common in males than females but this is reversed in Japan. In Europe and North America the inheritance appears to be polygenic or multifactorial. In the Middle East an autosomal recessive inheritance is apparent.

On gonioscopic examination several abnormalities are seen.

1 Abnormalities of iris insertion:
   (a) flat iris insertion with the iris inserting into the trabecular meshwork either anterior or posterior to the scleral spur;
   (b) concave iris insertion where the anterior stromal iris appears to continue over the trabecular meshwork obscuring the ciliary body and scleral spur.
2 Absent or rudimentary spur.
3 Wide open angle.
4 Normal Schlemm's canal.
5 Occasional iris process.
6 Amorphous tissue with vessels running from iris to Schwalbe's line (Barkan's membrane) (Fig. 15.3).

Usually, goniotomy or trabeculotomy is the accepted initial procedure for managing the elevated intraocular pressure.

Iridotrabeculodysgenesis
Axenfeld–Rieger anomaly
The term posterior embryotoxon is used to describe an abnormal thickening and anterior displacement of Schwalbe's line. The Axenfeld–Rieger anomaly is accompanied by:
- iridocorneal adhesions;
- high iris insertion on the trabecular meshwork obscuring the scleral spur;
- iris defects including stromal thinning, atrophy, corectopia and ectropion uveae (Fig. 15.4).

Glaucoma occurs in approximately 60% of these patients.

Rieger's syndrome
When systemic abnormalities accompany the above

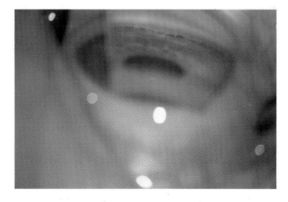

Fig. 15.3 Goniophotograph in primary congenital glaucoma. Schwalbe's line is barely visible anterior to the grey band of the iris insertion, posterior to which pigment knuckles project anteriorly from the iris root through bands of fine tissue extending from the anterior surface of the iris—'Barkan's membrane'.

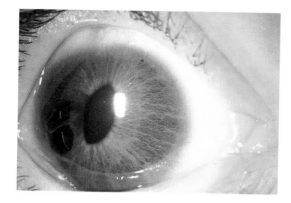

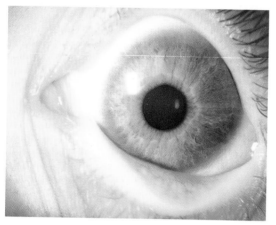

Fig. 15.4 Anterior segment dysgenesis. Bilateral glaucoma and Rieger's anomaly, more marked in the left eye.

ocular findings the term Rieger's syndrome has been used. These systemic abnormalities include:
• midface hypoplasia;
• telecanthus with a broad flat nasal root;
• dental anomalies — absent maxillary incisors, microdontia, anodontia;
• umbilical hernia;
• congenital heart anomalies;
• middle ear deafness;
• mental retardation;
• cerebellar vermis hypoplasia.

Although autosomal dominant inheritance with variable expressivity has been determined, the precise genetic defect has not yet been determined. Abnormalities of chromosomes 4, 6, 11 and 18 have

all been reported in association with Rieger's syndrome.

Aniridia (see Chapter 13)

This is a rare congenital bilateral anomaly that occurs in two distinct separate varieties: sporadic and autosomal dominantly inherited. Glaucoma occurs in more than 50% of affected individuals. The pathophysiology of the glaucoma appears to be variable. In some cases an anomalous angle without peripheral anterior synechiae is present and in others a progressive development of synechiae over time may lead to a secondary angle-closure glaucoma.

Syndromes associated with childhood glaucoma

A number of congenital disorders present with malformations of the anterior segment of the eye involving the cornea angle, iris and lens. Glaucoma may occur in some of these disorders.

Sturge–Weber syndrome (facial naevus flammeus)

(See Chapter 24.) This syndrome consists of the classic triad of:
1 portwine facial telangiectasis;
2 intracranial angiomas;
3 glaucoma (Fig. 15.5).

Approximately one-third of patients with the Sturge–Weber syndrome will develop glaucoma; in almost all cases it is unilateral. The glaucoma may occur in infancy but in many cases it does not develop until later in childhood. The pathophysiology of the glaucoma is variable and appears to be related to a developmental anomaly similar

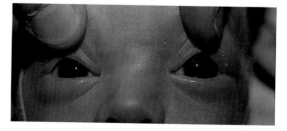

Fig. 15.5 Sturge–Weber syndrome with ipsilateral glaucoma.

to primary infantile glaucoma, raised episcleral venous pressure and premature ageing of the angle structures. Additional findings include choroidal haemangiomas that may increase the risk of choroidal detachment or haemorrhage during intraocular surgery. This disorder is sporadic with only a rare familial case having been reported.

Cutis marmorata telangiectasia congenita

This is a rare syndrome with many features in common with Sturge–Weber syndrome. It is a vascular disorder associated with a skin lesion referred to livedo reticularis, stroke-like episodes, seizures and glaucoma.

Neurofibromatosis

Glaucoma may occur in association with neurofibromatosis type 1. When it does, it is often associated with ipsilateral iris ectropion or lid and orbital plexiform neuromas. The aetiology of the glaucoma appears to be a combination of factors including abnormal tissue within the angle as well as angle closures secondary to neurofibromas.

Rubinstein–Taybi syndrome

This is a rare syndrome characterized by hypertelorism, antimongoloid slant, ptosis, long eyelashes, broad thumbs and great toes (Fig. 15.6). Glaucoma may be an associated finding presumably as the result of an underdevelopment of the angle.

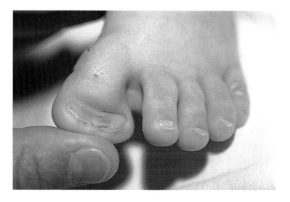

Fig. 15.6 Rubinstein–Taybi syndrome. Broad thumbs and toes are a characteristic feature.

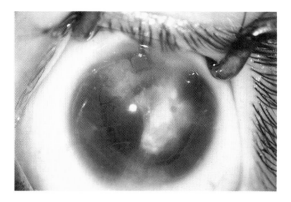

Fig. 15.7 Anterior segment dysgenesis with glaucoma (Peter's anomaly). Corneal opacities, to the posterior surface of which are attached iris strands. There is a cataract hidden by the corneal opacities.

Peter's anomaly

Peter's anomaly is defined as a congenital central corneal opacity with corresponding defects in the posterior corneal stroma, Descemet's membrane and endothelium (see Chapter 11). Glaucoma may be present at birth in association with Peter's anomaly or may occur following penetrating keratoplasty (Fig. 15.7).

Juvenile open-angle glaucoma

This autosomal dominantly inherited form of glaucoma is rare. Linkage to markers on 1q have been demonstrated. The clinical examination is unremarkable and gonioscopy does not show any abnormalities of the angle. Histopathological examination has isolated pathology in the trabecular meshwork.

Secondary glaucomas

Aphakic glaucoma

Glaucoma occurs in as many as 20–30% of patients following paediatric cataract surgery. The onset may be delayed for many years. The pathogenesis is not fully understood, although in some cases it appears to be related to associated developmental angle anomalies. Some authorities have associated it with specific cataract types, including nuclear cataracts and persistent hyperplastic vitreous (PHPV). Microphthalmos appears to be a significant risk factor. To what degree the surgical procedure itself is responsible is not certain. Treatment is usually difficult and the prognosis poor.

Retinopathy of prematurity

(See Chapter 17.) Glaucoma may occur even in severe retinopathy of prematurity with total retinal detachment. Mechanisms responsible seem to be multiple, including neovascular, angle closure and iridopupillary block.

Abnormal lens, iris diaphragm interaction

Patients with spherophakia (small spherical lenses) are prone to anterior dislocation and glaucoma. This may occur in isolated spherophakia or in the Weill–Marchesani syndrome. Although lenses in homocystinuria are of normal size, they have a propensity for anterior dislocation and associated glaucoma (Fig. 15.8).

Juvenile xanthogranuloma

Juvenile xanthogranulomas are benign lesions that commonly are seen on the skin and less commonly are associated with intraocular lesions that may lead to glaucoma. The glaucoma is most commonly secondary to bleeding (Fig. 15.9).

Glaucoma in inflammatory eye disease

Glaucoma can occur secondary to uveitis. Treatment is aimed at controlling the inflammation. The glaucoma may be the result of an acute trabeculitis or

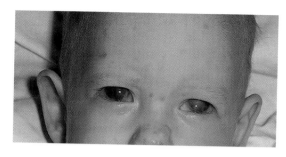

Fig. 15.9 Bilateral juvenile xanthogranuloma. Repeated haemorrhages gave rise to an intractable glaucoma in both eyes. Low-dose radiotherapy or topical steroids usually brings about rapid resolution of the condition.

inflammatory debris blocking the meshwork (see Chapter 13).

Trauma

Glaucoma may be associated with blunt trauma to the eye. It may occur with:
- hyphaema—the blood directly clogs the trabecular mesh;
- angle recession—usually produces a late onset of glaucoma.

Management of glaucoma in childhood

Decreased visual function in these patients occurs as the result of optic nerve damage, corneal opacification, cataracts and amblyopia. The problem of amblyopia cannot be overemphasised. It is frequently overlooked and not aggressively treated.

Clinical assessment of glaucoma

In the young child many of the standard assessment tools for the glaucoma patient cannot be utilized in the out-patient setting. Computerized perimetry is rarely possible in the preschool child, intraocular pressure measurements may be difficult to obtain in the office and corneal opacification and scarring may make examination of the optic nerve difficult. It is often necessary, therefore, to perform examinations under anaesthesia in order to fully assess the child with glaucoma.

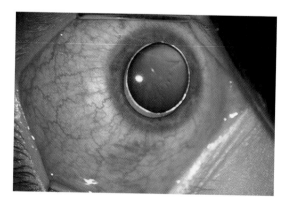

Fig. 15.8 Homocystinuria. Dislocated lens blocking the pupil and giving rise to glaucoma.

Box 15.1 The examination under anaesthesia (EUA) for glaucoma in infancy

Anaesthetic or sedation
Very small babies may not need any anaesthesia or sedation. Ketamine, suxamethonium and intubation tend to raise intraocular pressure. Halothane and many other agents lower intraocular pressure.

Parameters measured
1 Intraocular pressure is measured under general anaesthesia as soon after induction as possible. It is not in any circumstances an accurate or reliable measurement and should not be used as the only parameter to assess glaucoma.
2 Horizontal (and vertical) corneal diameter from limbus to limbus. This may be difficult in greatly expanded eyes where the limbus is indistinct.
3 Examination of the cornea for splits in Descemet's membrane and general clarity.
4 Refraction. Increasing myopia may reflect increasing eye size.
5 Eye volume by ultrasound.
6 Examination of the optic disc, estimation of the cup to disc ratio and comment on the state of the neural rim.

*It is preferable to make all measurements without reference to the previous notes to avoid bias

Therapy

Medical treatment

In most forms of glaucoma in children medical therapy is of only limited value. It is often used in an effort to stabilize intraocular pressure prior to surgery. A common combination is acetazolamide orally or intravenously, betaxolol and pilocarpine. The dosages used vary but should strictly be in milligrams per kilogram. A number of different surgical procedures have been developed for the treatment of glaucoma in children.

Goniotomy

This procedure is especially effective in treating trabeculodysgenesis. It does require a clear cornea;

corneal splits may therefore obscure the view and, if so, a trabeculotomy should be performed.

Yttrium–aluminium–garnet (YAG) laser goniotomy

Whether this procedure will produce long-term control comparable to surgical goniotomy is not yet known.

Trabeculotomy

This is the preferred procedure in the treatment of primary congenital glaucoma when a good view of the angle is not possible.

Combined trabeculotomy–trabeculectomy

This procedure may be particularly suited for the eye in which both abnormal angle and other ocular anomalies exist.

Trabeculectomy

There is a great tendency for filtration blebs to fail in young people. The introduction of 5-fluorouracil (5-FU), mitomycin and local radiotherapy have increased bleb survival.

Cyclocryotherapy

Ablation of the aqueous-producing ciliary body is utilised in cases where other surgical procedures have failed.

Cyclolaser therapy

This has a similar indication as cyclocryotherapy.

Endolaser

Endolaser has also been used with good effect.

Drainage tube implantation (setons)

A number of different forms of drainage tube implantation devices are now available. They are usually not used as the primary surgical procedure but only after other procedures have failed. The complication of early hypotony has been reduced with refinement of the drainage devices and improved surgical techniques.

16: Vitreous

Development

The primary vitreous appears at approximately 6 weeks' gestation and is composed of mesodermal cells, collagenous fibrillary material, hyaloid vessels and macrophages. The secondary vitreous forms at approximately 2 months and contains compact fibrillary network, hyalocytes, monocytes and a small amount of hyaluronic acid. At the end of the third month the tertiary vitreous forms as a thickened accumulation of collagen fibres between the lens equator and optic cup. This is the precursor to the vitreous base and lens zonules. Towards the end of the fourth month of gestation the primary vitreous and hyaloid vasculature atrophies to become a clear narrow central zone that is referred to as Cloquet's canal. Persistence of the primary vitreous is important in a number of developmental anomalies of the vitreous.

Developmental anomalies

Persistent hyaloid artery

Persistence of the hyaloid artery may be seen in upwards of 3% of normal full-term infants. It is seen almost universally in 30-week gestational age or younger prematures when screening for retinopathy of prematurity. Posterior remnants of this hyaloid system may appear as an elevated mass of glial tissue on the disc and is referred to as Bergmeister's papilla. An anterior remnant seen adherent to the posterior lens capsule is referred to as Mittendorf's dot.

Persistent hyperplastic vitreous (PHPV)

PHPV is a congenital abnormality of the eye caused by failure of the primary vitreous to regress. It is usually sporadic and unilateral. Many of the cases reported to be bilateral and familial probably represent examples of various syndromes with vitreoretinal dysplasia. The classic features of PHPV include:
- fibrous plaque adherent to the back of the lens;
- microphthalmos;
- shallow anterior chamber;
- dilated iris vessels;
- vascularised retrolental membrane with traction on the ciliary processes (Fig. 16.1).

Other ocular associations with PHPV seen infrequently include:
- megalocornea;
- Rieger's anomaly;
- morning glory disc anomaly.

Although a so-called posterior PHPV form has been described it is not clear in what way these cases differ from falciform folds or vitreoretinal dysplasias.

Treatment of PHPV is usually directed to preventing glaucoma and phthisis bulbi. Removal of the lens and posterior membrane may prevent glaucoma even in an eye in which the visual prognosis is poor. However, it should be noted that glaucoma has been reported even after lensectomy–vitrectomy. Occasional reports have documented good visual acuity with early surgery and aggressive anti-amblyopic therapy.

Vitreous cysts

Cysts of the vitreous may be either congenital or acquired (Fig. 16.2). The origin of the cysts is unknown but since blood vessels are sometimes seen within congenital cysts the possibility that they have their origin from hyaloid artery remnants has been suggested.

Acquired cysts may be seen in association with:
- toxoplasmosis;
- toxocariasis;
- juvenile retinoschisis.

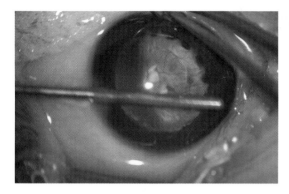

Fig. 16.1 PHPV with a vascularized retrolental membrane. There was a large persistent hyaloid artery. If removed sufficiently early, and optically corrected together with occlusion of the fellow eye, useful acuity may sometimes be salvaged.

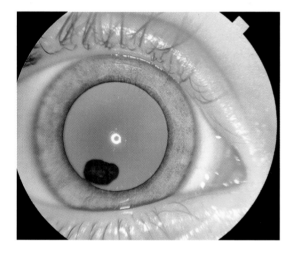

Fig. 16.2 Anterior vitreous cyst seen in retroillumination. The acuity was 6/5 and the eye otherwise healthy.

Vitreoretinal dysplasia

Vitreoretinal dysplasia may be seen as an isolated ocular anomaly or in association with a variety of systemic abnormalities (Fig. 16.3).

Trisomy 13 (Patau's syndrome)

Bilateral severe ocular abnormalities occur in almost all cases of trisomy 13 and include the following:

- extensive retinal dysplasia;
- intraocular cartilage;
- microphthalmos;
- colobomas;
- cyclopia;
- cataracts;
- corneal opacities;
- glaucoma.

Severe systemic abnormalities are also found and preclude prolonged survival.

Norrie's disease (Andersen–Warburg disease)

Norrie's disease is an X-linked recessive disorder in which blindness, deafness and mental retardation may occur. At least three affected females with severe visual loss have been reported. The gene for Norrie's disease has been identified and it encodes a protein with 133 amino acids. Deletions or additions of residues of this gene have been identified in affected families.

Identification of the Norrie's disease gene will permit diagnosis of the carrier state and diagnosis of the affected individual.

Ocular findings include:

- bilateral retinal folds;
- retinal detachment;
- vitreous haemorrhage;
- bilateral retrolental masses (vitreoretinal dysplasia);
- phthisis bulbi (Fig. 16.4).

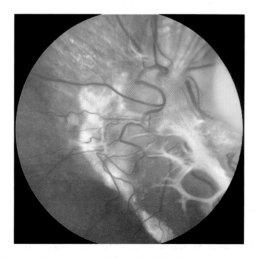

Fig. 16.3 An extensive vitreoretinal dysplasia.

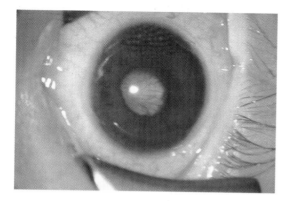

Fig. 16.4 Norrie's disease showing vascularized white retrolental mass.

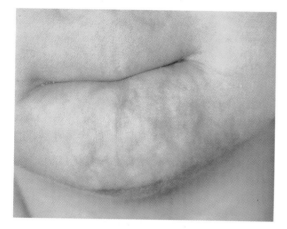

Fig. 16.5 Incontinentia pigmenti showing pigmented skin lesions of the chin.

Almost all affected males are blind at birth or in early infancy. Approximately 25% of affected males are mentally retarded and 33% develop cochlear hearing loss.

Incontinentia pigmenti (Bloch–Sulzberger syndrome)

This is a rare disorder involving ectodermal structures (such as eyes, skin, teeth and central nervous system). Affected patients usually present in infancy with a vesicular eruption of the skin that evolves into a whirling pattern of abnormal pigmentation. This becomes less apparent with age (Fig. 16.5). It is inherited as an X-linked dominant

('male lethal') syndrome and has been mapped by linkage studies to the Xq28 region. No male-to-male transmission has been documented, although male-to-female transmission has.

Ocular abnormalities include:
• retinal vascular abnormalities—vascular tortuosity, capillary closure, peripheral or venous shunts;
• preretinal fibrosis;
• traction retinal detachment;
• retinal haemorrhages;
• macular oedema;
• cataract;
• optic atrophy;
• nystagmus and strabismus.

Treatment of the affected female with cryotherapy or photocoagulation as soon as the retinal vascular abnormalities are identified may prevent retinal detachment.

Walker–Warburg syndrome (hardA +/−E)

This is an autosomal recessive syndrome with:
• vitreoretinal dysplasia and lissencephaly (agyria);
• cerebellar malformation;
• congenital muscular dystrophy;
• Dandy–Walker malformation;
• encephalocoele (Fig. 16.6).

Other vitreoretinal dysplasia syndromes include:
• osteoporosis with pseudoglioma
  (a) mental retardation
  (b) inherited as autosomal recessive disorder;
• oculo-palato-cerebral dwarfism
  (a) microcephaly
  (b) mental retardation
  (c) cleft palate
  (d) short stature
  (e) associated with findings that resemble PHPV either unilaterally or bilaterally.

Inherited vitreoretinal degeneration and retinal detachment

Stickler's syndrome (hereditary progressive arthro-ophthalmopathy)

Stickler described a syndrome consisting of high myopia and early retinal detachment associated

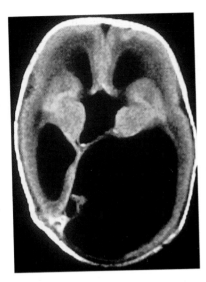

Fig. 16.6 Walker–Warburg syndrome. Computerized tomography scan showing hydrocephalus, lissencephaly and colpocephaly. Occipital encephalocoeles are present in some cases.

with premature degenerative changes of the articular cartilage. It is inherited as an autosomal dominant trait and in some reports appears to be more common than Marfan's syndrome. The ocular features include:

- congenital stable high myopia;
- syneretic vitreous;
- vitreous membranes and veils;
- perivascular pigmentary changes of the retina;
- chorioretinal degeneration and retinal breaks;
- primary open-angle glaucoma;
- presenile nuclear cataracts;
- peripheral cortical cataracts—'spoke-like'.
  Systemic abnormalities include:
- progressive arthropathy;
- cleft palate and lip;
- abnormal facial features;
- sensory neural hearing loss.

This is a clinically heterogeneous group of dominant disorders of several subtypes, including a marfanoid variant, a variant with the Pierre–Robin anomaly and patients with the more classic phenotype of a flattened face and depressed bridge of the nose. The gene for one form of Stickler's syndrome has been mapped to 12q14. More recent mutations have been identified to COL2AI. These patients need to be carefully examined and prophylactic treatment for any retinal holes with cryotherapy or laser is recommended. Management of the retinal detachments is complex and often not successful.

Kniest's syndrome

This syndrome is closely related to the Stickler's syndrome and is also inherited as an autosomal dominant trait. Systemic abnormalities associated with this syndrome include:

- bone dysplasia;
- prominent wide joints;
- short trunk;
- protrusion of the sternum;
- flat midface with depressed nasal bridge;
- cleft palate.
  Ocular features include:
- high myopia;
- cataract;
- glaucoma;
- retinal detachment.
  Treatment is similar to the Stickler's syndrome.

Wagner's syndrome

This is an isolated ocular syndrome with no systemic manifestations. Its ocular features include:

- moderate myopia;
- optically empty vitreous;
- preretinal avascular membrane;
- retinal vascular changes with sheathing and perivascular pigmentation;
- progressive retinal and choroidal atrophy;
- progressive retinal degeneration that may progress to an extinguished electroretinogram (ERG);
- no retinal detachment;
- cataracts.

This syndrome has been linked to 5q13–q14. The prognosis in this syndrome is usually good with a very slow progression of the retinal dystrophy.

Juvenile X-linked retinoschisis (congenital hereditary retinoschisis)

This disorder that has no systemic manifestations is inherited as an X-linked recessive trait. The abnormal gene has been localized to the Xp22 region.

Affected female carriers exhibit no abnormalities. Its ocular features include the following.

• Foveal retinoschisis—occurs in 50% of cases and is the most constant finding; may be seen even in early infancy (Fig. 16.7). Visual acuity usually is in the range of 6/12–6/36.

• Inferotemporal retinoschisis—seen in 40–50% of patients. A split appears in the nerve fibre layer; bleeding may occur from bridging vessels (Fig. 16.8) which break leading to vitreous haemorrhage.

• Vitreous veils (fibrous condensation of vitreous cortex) — usually over the areas of peripheral retinoschisis.

• Posterior vitreous detachment.

• Pigmentary retinopathy, perivascular sheathing, capillary closure.

• Abnormal ERG showing a reduced or abnormal B wave in the presence of a normal A wave.

This is considered to be an abnormality of Mueller cells causing both the macular and peripheral retinal changes.

Goldmann–Favre disease

This is a rare autosomal recessive condition with no systemic manifestations. Ocular features include:

• retinoschisis;

• progressive cataract;

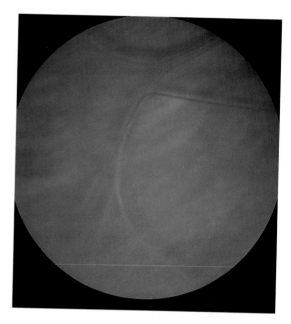

Fig. 16.8 Juvenile X-linked retinoschisis. Peripheral schisis with vessels visible in the schitic strands. Vitreous haemorrhage is not uncommon.

• pigmentary chorioretinal degeneration;

• liquefaction of the vitreous;

• microcystic macular changes.

Visual loss is primarily related to macular schisis and occurs early in the disease, with 6/36 visual acuity not uncommon in childhood.

Familial exudative vitreoretinopathy (FEVR)

FEVR is a term used to describe a group of inherited disorders characterized by abnormal retinal vascularisation in association with exudation, neovascularisation and tractional retinal detachment. The clinical appearance may mimic retinopathy of prematurity. Almost certainly some reported cases of retinopathy of prematurity occurring in non-premature infants were caused by this disorder. Two primary forms exist.

1 Autosomal dominant form—mapped to the long arm of chromosome 11.

2 X-linked recessive form — mapped to either Xp21.3 or Xp11; may be allelic with Norrie's disease.

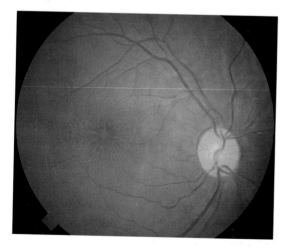

Fig. 16.7 Juvenile X-linked retinoschisis showing foveal star-shaped retinoschisis.

Autosomal dominant exudative vitreoretinopathy

No systemic abnormalities are associated with this progressive vitreoretinopathy in which the most constant ocular finding is an abrupt termination of retinal vessels along a scalloped edge at the equator of the retina. However, there is a wide range of clinical expression even amongst members of the same family.

The ocular features of this disorder include:
- peripheral retinovascular abnormalities (Fig. 16.9)
   - (a) vascular dilatation
   - (b) tortuosity
   - (c) arteriovenous shunting
   - (d) capillary closure
   - (e) peripheral neovascularization;
- optic disc neovascularization;
- macular ectopia;
- tractional retinal detachment;
- macular oedema;
- subretinal exudate.

The majority of retinal detachments occur in the first decade of life and very little progression of this disease occurs after the age of 10 years.

X-linked FEVR

This rare disorder may be indistinguishable from severe forms of dominant exudative vitreoretinopathy. It is characterized by an early onset and usually poor prognosis. It may be allelic with Norrie's disease.

Autosomal dominant vitreoretinochoroidopathy (ADVIRC)

This condition is characterized by an abnormal chorioretinal hypopigmentation and hyperpigmentation found between the vortex veins and the ora serrata for 360°. A distinct posterior border appears near the equator. Cystoid macular oedema or vitreous haemorrhage may occur in children as young as the age of 7 years. No systemic abnormalities are seen in this disorder. Ocular abnormalities include:
- retinovascular changes
   - (a) retinal arterial narrowing
   - (b) venous occlusion
   - (c) widespread vascular leakage;
- diffuse liquefaction of the vitreous;
- presenile cataract;
- macular oedema;
- vitreous haemorrhage and retinal detachment;
- ERG is normal in most individuals;
- EOG is usually abnormal.

Autosomal dominant neovascular inflammatory vitreoretinopathy (ADNIV)

This rare autosomal dominant disorder is characterized by retinal vascular occlusion and neovascularization which may lead to vitreous haemorrhage and tractional retinal detachment. The gene responsible has recently been mapped to chromosome 11q13. Unlike ADVIRC, this is a progressive disorder in which selective loss of the B wave on ERG testing may be seen. Up to 20% of affected individuals develop retinal detachments.

Erosive vitreoretinopathy

This is an autosomal dominant disorder characterized by:
- nyctalopia;
- progressive visual field loss;
- vitreous abnormalities;
- progressive retinal pigment atrophy;
- retinal detachment;

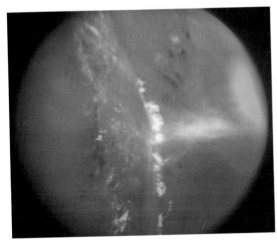

Fig. 16.9 Dominant exudative vitreoretinopathy showing preretinal and retinal vascular changes.

- widespread rod/cone dysfunction seen on ERG test.

The visual prognosis is poor; retinal detachment occurs in most affected adults.

Autosomal dominant snowflake degeneration (hereditary snowflake vitreoretinal degeneration of Hirose)

This disorder is named because of the presence of white snowflake-like spots that are 100–200 μm in size and appear in areas of 'white with pressure'. These are not usually seen in the first two decades of life. Four ophthalmoscopically distinct stages have been described.

1 Stage I. Extensive 'white with pressure'.
2 Stage II. Snowflake-like spots extending from the equator to the ora serrata.
3 Stage III. Sheathing of retinal vessels in the area of snowflake degeneration.
4 Stage IV. Increased pigmentary changes in the area of snowflake degeneration.

As this disorder progresses, constriction of visual field, elevation of rod thresholds in dark adaptation and decrease in amplitude of the scotopic B wave are noted. There are no associated systemic abnormalities.

Acquired disorders of the vitreous

Inflammatory disease of the vitreous

Vitreous inflammatory disease in childhood may include all of the following:
- juvenile pars planitis;
- intermediate uveitis;
- retinal vasculitis;
- juvenile rheumatoid arthritis;
- sarcoidosis;
- tuberculosis;
- toxoplasmosis;
- toxocariasis;
- acute retinal necrosis.

Although bacterial infection involving the vitreous is uncommon in childhood, it may occur in three distinct settings.

1 Following ocular surgery (including strabismus surgery).
2 Following penetrating trauma.
3 Endogenous metastatic endophthalmitis — seen in association with acquired immune deficiency syndrome (AIDS), in the immunologically compromised patient, and meningitis.

Tumour seeding of the vitreous

Vitreous seeding is a common finding in retinoblastoma. It may also occur in leukaemia. Other causes are extremely rare.

Box 16.1 Vitreous haemorrhage

Vitreous haemorrhage may occur in a wide range of disorders that include:
- PHVP;
- X-linked juvenile retinoschisis;
- FEVR, ADVIRC, ADNIV—secondary to neovascularization;
- Stickler's syndrome;
- retinal haemangioblastomas;
- cavernous haemangioma;
- Eale's disease;
- Coats' disease;
- bleeding diathesis.

In most cases conservative management of vitreous haemorrhage is indicated, although in the amblyogenic period vitrectomy may be necessary if form deprivation amblyopia appears to be a risk.

17: Retina

Retinal vascular anomalies and diseases

Retinal haemangiomas

Retinal capillary haemangiomas
These angiomas are found most frequently in von Hippel–Lindau disease (see Chapter 24):
- peripapillary;
- peripheral;
- fluorescein angiography may identify subclinical lesions;
- present with visual symptoms or found during routine examination;
- treatment mandatory with photocoagulation or cryotherapy, larger peripheral tumours treated with radiotherapy or scleral radioactive plaque.

Retinal cavernous haemangiomas
- Congenital or early onset.
- Bright red, grape-like clusters.
- Slow blood flow (Fig. 17.1).
- Spontaneous improvement occurs, haemorrhage rare.
- Treatment with laser or cryotherapy if haemorrhages are recurrent.

Racemose haemangiomas
- Large retinal veins.
- Arteriovenous anastamosis frequent.
- Vision often relatively good.
- Treatment unnecessary.
- May be associated with intracranial vascular malformation (Wyburn–Mason's syndrome) (Fig. 17.2)

Retinal vascular anomalies (see Chapter 18)
- Cilioretinal arteries.
- Persistent hyaloid arteries.
- Prepapillary vascular loops.

- Myelinated nerve fibres.
- Fundus colobomas.
- Aicardi's syndrome.

Coats' disease
In Coats' disease there are congenital retinal telangiectases which lead to subretinal fluid accumulation and an exudative retinal detachment. It usually occurs in boys (3 : 1), is mostly unilateral and is diagnosed by the finding of aneurysmal dilatation of peripheral vessels together with subretinal exudation which is not calcified (Fig. 17.3).

Treatment with light or laser photocoagulation or cryotherapy to the telangiectatic vessels may reduce the exudation but this treatment may bring about vitreous haemorrhage. A similar condition occurs in:
- facio-scapulo-humeral muscular dystrophy;
- other muscular dystrophies;
- hemifacial atrophy;
- congenital plasminogen deficiency;
- others (see D. Taylor (ed.), Chapter 46, *Paediatric Ophthalmology,* 2nd edn, 1997, Blackwell Science, Oxford).

Diabetic retinopathy
- Older children only. The risk of diabetic retinopathy increases with the years after diagnosis.
- Retinal oedema and mild background retinopathy; the most common abnormality in childhood.

Retinal vasculitis
In this, there is a retinal vascular inflammation with vessels sheathing, beading, haemorrhages, exudates and signs of occlusion such as cotton wool spots (Fig. 17.4) and neovascularization. There is associated posterior uveitis and vitritis.
1 Eale's disease:
   (a) young men or older children;

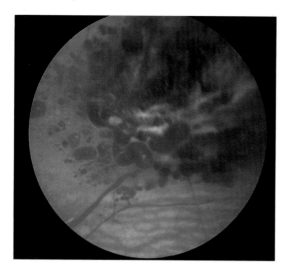

Fig. 17.1 Cavernous haemangioma of the retina. This 11-month-old child presented with a squint, but with patching the eye the acuity remained at 6/18. The grape-like cluster of abnormal vessels was adjacent to the macular and regressed over 3 years.

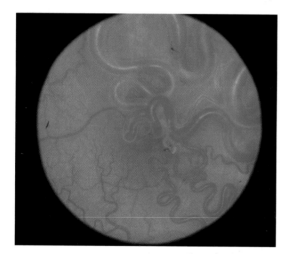

Fig. 17.2 Congenital retinal macro vessels. The acuity was 6/18.

   (b) peripheral, bilateral small vessel closure;
   (c) frond-like neovascularization and haemor-rhage;
   (d) associated with tuberculosis.
2 Systemic lupus erythematosus, etc.
3 Sarcoidosis—peripheral sheathed veins.

4 Idiopathic retinal vasculitis.
5 Behçet's disease.
6 Frosted branch periphlebitis:
   (a) rare;
   (b) unilateral;
   (c) visual loss;
   (d) uveitis;
   (e) marked venous sheathing.
7 Macular oedema and exudative serous detach-ment—good prognosis.

Cystoid macular oedema

Cystoid macular oedema, which on fluorescein angiogram shows a star-shaped intraretinal lesion caused by leakage from perifoveolar capillaries.

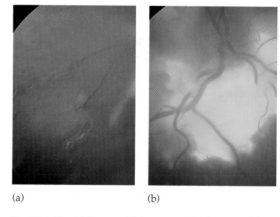

(a)   (b)

Fig. 17.3 Coats' disease. (a) Aneurysmal dilatation of the retinal arterioles. (b) Exudative retinal detachment with subretinal solid exudate.

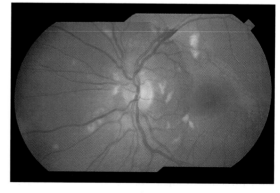

Fig. 17.4 Retinal vasculitis in systemic lupus erythematosus showing multiple cotton wool spots.

- Retinal vasculitis.
- Uveitis and pars planitis.
- Retinal and macular dystrophies.
- May be idiopathic and autosomal dominantly inherited.
- Following any retinal vasculopathy.
- Possibly following infant cataract surgery.

Pigment epithelial and other retinal lesions

Grouped pigmentation (bear-track pigmentation)
- Unilateral.
- Multiple pigmented lesions in retinal pigment epithelium (Fig. 17.4).
- Benign, non-progressive.

Congenital hypertrophy of the retinal pigment epithelium (CHRPE)
- Solitary, well-defined black retinal pigment epithelial (RPE) lesions.
- One to two disc diameters, may have depigmented halo.
- Fluorescein shows masking by the CHRPE.
- Isolated without systemic involvement.
- Associated with:
  (a) familial adenomatous polyposis coli—the individuals who carry the gene for familial adenomatous polyposis coli—there are usually more than three CHRPE lesions in the two eyes;
  (b) autosomal dominant;
  (c) colonic polyps with malignant potential;
  (d) with osteomas, desmoid tumours and epidermoid cysts—Gardner's syndrome;
  (e) with neuroepithelial and central nervous system tumours—Turcot's syndrome.

Combined hamartoma of the retina and RPE
These are lesions usually around the optic discs which are raised, contain pigment and tortuous and beaded vessels (Fig. 17.5). They are slowly progressive and may affect vision by macular involvement. They present often in young children with strabismus or are occasionally found on routine fundus examination. Since they are frequently found in

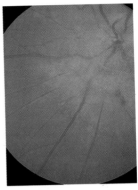

Fig. 17.5 Combined hamartoma of the retina and retinal pigment epithelium. There is elevation of the optic disc with radial retinal traction and a wrinkled internal limiting membrane with RPE changes around the optic disc.

neurofibromatosis type 2, affected patients should be screened for this condition.

Epiretinal membranes
These are rare in childhood and present with strabismus or visual distortion. A diaphanous membrane is seen on the surface of the retina distorting blood vessels and the macula.

Aetiology
- Idiopathic.
- Post-traumatic.
- Diabetes (rare in children).
- Associated with neurofibromatosis type 2.

In children with no other abnormality and no history of trauma the finding of an epiretinal membrane should lead to a search for neurofibromatosis type 2.

Lamellar macular holes
These are partial thickness macular holes with vision variably, not markedly reduced.
- Idiopathic.
- Post-traumatic.
- Following cystoid macular oedema.

Retinal phakoma
- Astrocytic hamartoma.
- Isolated or associated with tuberous sclerosis.

- Mostly at the posterior pole.
- Calcification shows on computerized tomography (CT) or ultrasound.
- Early translucent masses near blood vessels.
- Later lesions knobbly, raised and opaque 'mulberry tumours'.
- Complicated by vitreous haemorrhages, glaucoma and retinal detachment.

Retinal detachment in children

Retinal detachment in childhood is difficult to manage because it is often diagnosed late, the child being asymptomatic unless the second eye is affected. Often there are severe underlying vitreoretinal conditions which carry a poor prognosis, and pre-operative assessment and postoperative management are difficult because of lack of co-operation in many children.

Surgical management of retinal detachment is the province of the specialist retinal surgeon.

Box 17.1 Retinal detachment in children

Rhegmatogenous
- Traumatic.
- Non-traumatic:
  (a) retinopathy of prematurity (ROP);
  (b) retinal dialysis.
- Marfan's syndrome.
- Spondyloepiphyseal dysplasia.
- Retinoschisis (see Chapter 16).
- Colobomas.
- Aphakic.
- Associated with myopia.

Non-rhegmatogenous
- ROP.
- Posterior uveitis (see Chapter 13).
- Familial exudative retinopathy (see Chapter 16).
- Incontinentia pigmenti.
- Optic disc pits.
- Coats' disease.
- Retinal tumours—retinoblastoma.
- Choroidal tumours—haemangiomas, etc.

Spondyloepiphyseal dysplasias

One of the more common and more difficult conditions to manage is Stickler's syndrome and other forms of spondyloepiphyseal dysplasia. These children have congenital high myopia which is generally non-progressive. It may be associated with cataract and there are dysmorphic features including midface hypoplasia, spine and joint changes (Fig. 17.6).

Management of retinal detachments in childhood

Retinal detachments in childhood often have a poor prognosis and need to be managed by an experienced vitreoretinal surgeon, preferably in a unit with access to paediatric services.

Retinopathy of prematurity (ROP)

Pathogenesis

Although this condition, which occurs predominantly in premature babies, was originally thought to be due to oxygen administration, the cause now appears to be multifactorial.

- *Gestational age (GA)*—the shorter the GA the more likely and the more severe the retinopathy is likely to be. The onset is most likely to be between 28 and 45 weeks. Infants of less than 28 weeks are rarely affected.
- *Birth weight*—ROP is unusual in infants weighing more than 1500 g; the incidence decreases as the birth weight increases.
- *Oxygen* — ROP is relatively infrequent when inspired air has up to 40% oxygen. Inspired oxygen concentration is normally adjusted by arterial or transcutaneous blood gas monitoring in most neonatal units
- Supplemental causative factors:
  (a) twins;
  (b) hypercarbia;
  (c) hypercapnia;
  (d) intraventricular haemorrhage;
  (e) repeated bradycardias;
  (f) recurrent apnoea;
  (g) respiratory distress syndrome;
  (h) lack of surfactant;
  (i) relative vitamin E deficiency;
  (j) exchange transfusions (use adult blood).

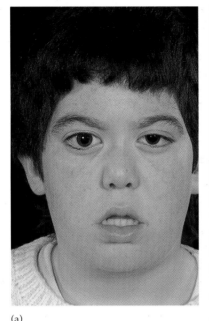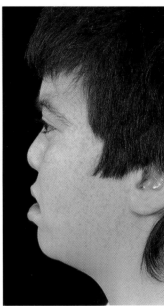

Fig. 17.6 Stickler's syndrome. (a) Vitreous opacities and strands. The vitreoretinal problems in these children makes them very susceptible to retinal detachment. (b) Showing the flat nasal bridge and midfacial hypoplasia and deafness (note hearing aid). Micrognathia, cleft palate and dental abnormalities may also be present.

(a)

(b)

International classification

Location

The retina is divided into three zones—one, two and three (Fig. 17.7).

- Zone one — centred on disc, two times disc–macular distance.
- Zone two — edge of zone one to ora serrata nasally, to the equator temporally.
- Zone three—all retina anterior to zone two.

Extent

In clock hours (see Fig. 17.7).

Natural history

Most stage I and II ROP resolve completely, sometimes associated with myopia. Some progress through stage III, most particularly children with low birth weight, shorter GA, oxygen usage and additional causative factors.

Ocular examination of the premature infant

1 Pupil dilatation:
  (a) cyclopentolate 0.5%;
  (b) phenylephrine 2.5%;

> **Box 17.2 Stages of severity**
>
> Stages of ROP (from the Committee for Classification of ROP, 1987).
> - Stage I—demarcation line (Fig. 17.8).
> - Stage II — ridge; a few neovascular tufts may be seen behind the ridge (Fig. 17.9).
> - Stage III—ridge with extraretinal neovascularization (Fig. 17.10).
> - Stage IV—subtotal retinal detachment:
>   (a) extrafoveal;
>   (b) foveal.
> - Stage V—total retinal detachment:
>   (a) open funnel;
>   (b) closed funnel (Fig. 17.11).
> - Plus disease (suggests progression):
>   (a) retinal and iris vascular dilatation;
>   (b) vitreous haze;
>   (c) difficulty in pupil dilatation.

  (c) both are given together 40 minutes prior to examination, and repeated at 15 and 30 minutes if necessary—lasts 4–6 hours.
2 Examination in the nursery or SCBU:
  (a) nurse assistant helpful;

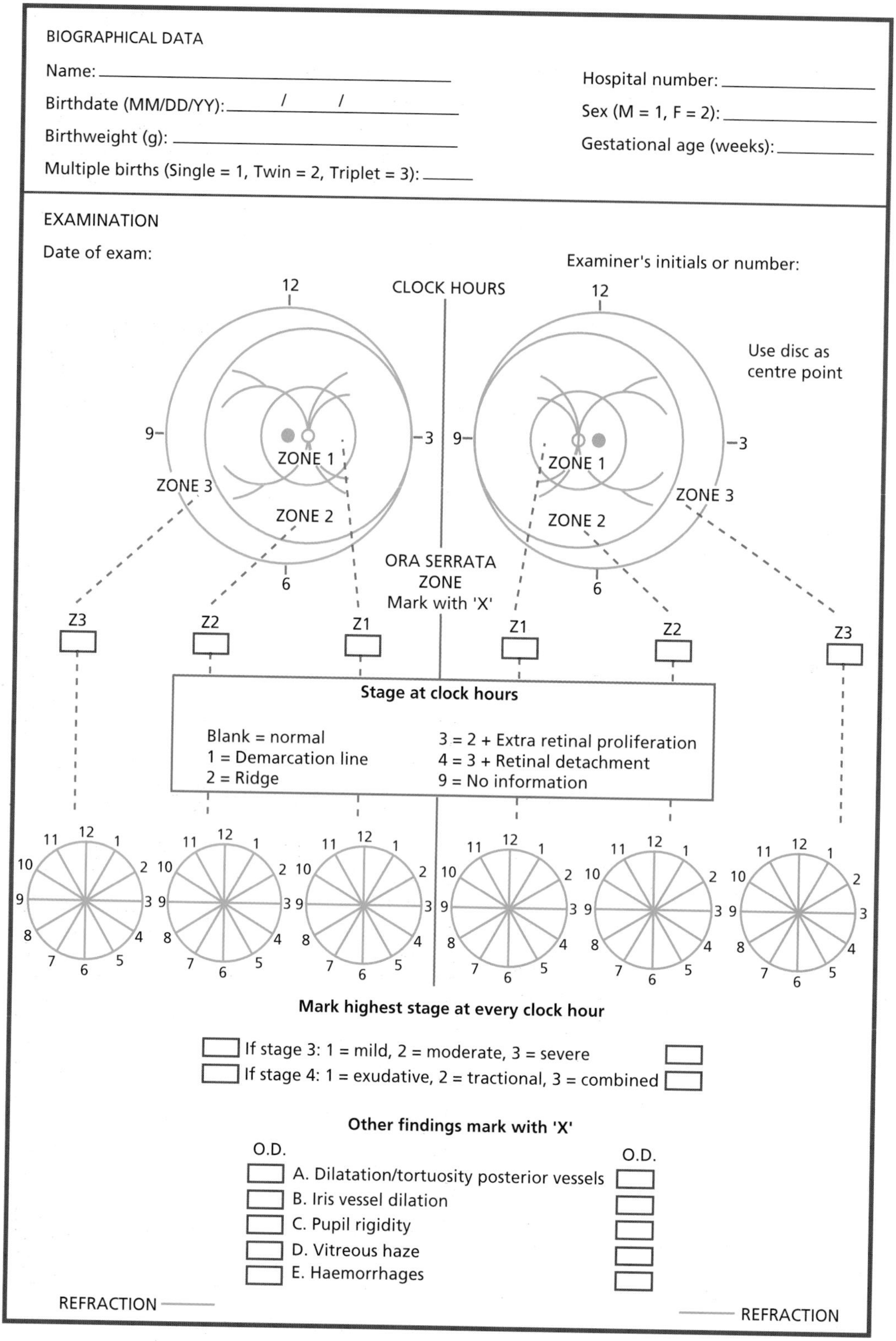

BIOGRAPHICAL DATA

Name: _____

Birthdate (MM/DD/YY): _____ / _____ / _____

Birthweight (g): _____

Multiple births (Single = 1, Twin = 2, Triplet = 3): _____

Hospital number: _____

Sex (M = 1, F = 2): _____

Gestational age (weeks): _____

EXAMINATION

Date of exam:

Examiner's initials or number: _____

CLOCK HOURS

Use disc as centre point

12   12

9—   —3 9—   —3

ZONE 1   ZONE 1

ZONE 3   ZONE 3

ZONE 2   ZONE 2

6   6

ORA SERRATA
ZONE
Mark with 'X'

Z3   Z2   Z1   Z1   Z2   Z3

Stage at clock hours

Blank = normal   3 = 2 + Extra retinal proliferation
1 = Demarcation line   4 = 3 + Retinal detachment
2 = Ridge   9 = No information

Mark highest stage at every clock hour

If stage 3: 1 = mild, 2 = moderate, 3 = severe
If stage 4: 1 = exudative, 2 = tractional, 3 = combined

Other findings mark with 'X'

O.D.   O.D.

A. Dilatation/tortuosity posterior vessels
B. Iris vessel dilation
C. Pupil rigidity
D. Vitreous haze
E. Haemorrhages

REFRACTION _____   _____ REFRACTION

Fig. 17.7 A chart for recording fundus details and staging ROP.

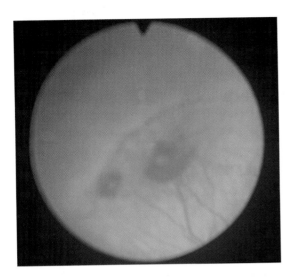

Fig. 17.8 ROP stage I demarcation line. The haemorrhages are perinatal and not related to the ROP.

4 Funduscopy using indirect ophthalmoscope with or without indentation. The role of the indenter is as much to move the eye as to indent the sclera. Caution must be used in interpreting fundus signs when indentation used. Lens of 28 or 20 D are used. The anterior segment should be examined using the indirect ophthalmoscope lens.

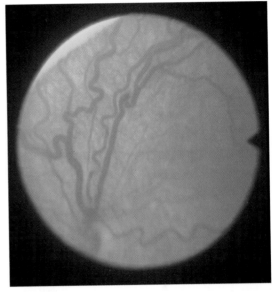

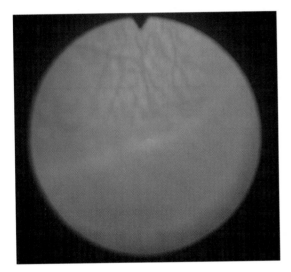

Fig. 17.9 ROP stage II ridge projecting (out of focus) forward into the vitreous.

(b) full monitoring of oxygen and heart—the procedure may need to be abandoned if the child becomes sick;
(c) speculum inserted after insertion of topical anaesthetic drop.
3 Refraction using lens rack and retinoscope.

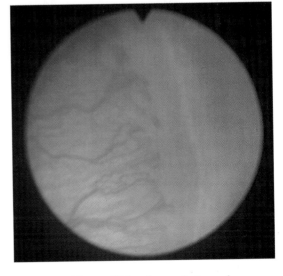

Fig. 17.10 ROP stage III showing marked vascular dilatation of tortuosity and a ridge with new vessels.

5 All clinical findings should be recorded pictorially or on a chart similar to that shown in Fig. 17.7 where possible.

Screening protocol

All infants of less than 1500 g and less than 32 weeks gestation need to be examined, whether or not they have been sick or have had prolonged or high levels of oxygen.

- Infants up to 26 weeks GA:
  (a) 7 weeks post-natally;
  (b) every 2 weeks until 36 weeks GA.
- Infants 26–32 weeks GA:
  (a) 7 weeks post-natally;
  (b) 36 weeks GA or at discharge from hospital around this time.

Follow-up as indicated by clinical criteria.

Treatment

Cryotherapy or laser treatment is used. The treatment threshold is: stage III, involving 5 contiguous or 8 cumulative clock hours in zones 3 or 2 and any disease in zone 1. If stage II with 'plus' disease is present in zone 2 this may also be an indication for treatment. Zone 1 involvement carries a very poor prognosis.

The aim of cryotherapy or laser treatment is to ablate the avascular retinal anterior to the ROP ridge, usually for 360°. Anaesthesia or sedation is usually used for cryotherapy.

Outcome

1 Regression.
2 Progression — especially if plus disease signs present.

Late complications of regressed ROP

- Myopia.
- Peripheral retinal scarring.
- Dragged retinal vessels.
- Dragged macular.
- Retinal folds.
- Strabismus.
- Associated central visual defects.
- Late retinal detachment.

Complications of stage V ROP

- Retinal fibrous.

- Retinal vitreous haemorrhage.
- Vitreous and retinal organisation and scarring.
- Retrolental membrane formation.
- Anterior thrusting of the lens/iris diaphragm giving rise to glaucoma, corneal decompensation and phthisis. This may require preventative lensectomy if the anterior chamber progressively flattens.

Retinal detachment and vitreous surgery in stage V ROP is generally unrewarding from the point of view of visual rehabilitation (Fig. 17.11).

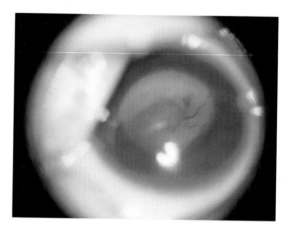

Fig. 17.11 ROP stage V. Funnel-shaped retinal detachment.

Retinoblastoma

Hereditary retinoblastoma

- Fifty per cent of all cases.
- Autosomal dominant, due to a mutation in both alleles of the *RB1* gene at 13q14.1–q14.2. Knudson's hypothesis was that there was a germ-line and a local mutation.
- Usually bilateral.
- Usually multifocal.
- Usually early onset.

Non-hereditary retinoblastoma

- *RB1* mutation in both alleles in a single primitive retinal cell.
- Unilateral.
- Monofocal, smaller.
- Later onset.

(Fifteen per cent of unilateral retinoblastoma patients have a germ-line (hereditary) *RB1* mutation.)

Other RB1 mutation defects

- Retinoma (Fig. 17.12):
  (a) benign retinal tumour;
  (b) white;
  (c) non-progressive or slowly progressive.
- Trilateral retinoblastoma:
  (a) bilateral retinoblastoma with pineal retinoblastoma;
  (b) hydrocephalus;
  (c) familial.
- Non-ocular malignancies:
  (a) osteosarcoma — orbital and remote, especially within the irradiation field;
  (b) others.
- Cytogenetically visible 13q14 deletions.
  (a) bilateral retinoblastoma;
  (b) mental retardation;
  (c) dysmorphism.

Presentation of retinoblastoma

1 Leucocoria.
2 Strabismus or poor vision.

3 Acute red eye from glaucoma or uveitis with tumour necrosis.
4 Orbital cellulitis.
5 Pupil or iris changes.
6 Hyphaema or hypopyon.
7 Mydriasis.

Box 17.3 Differential diagnosis of leucocoria

1 Retinoblastoma.
2 *Toxocara.*
3 Coats' disease.
4 Retinal dysplasia, Norrie's, autosomal recessive, Warburg's syndrome.
5 Cataract.
6 Persistent hyperplastic vitreous (PHPV).
7 ROP.
8 Endophthalmitis.
9 Medulloepithelioma.
10 Myelinated nerve fibres.
11 Coloboma and morning glory syndrome.
12 Chronic uveitis, toxocariasis or intermediate uveitis.
13 Vitreous haemorrhage.
14 Dominant exudative vitreoretinopathy.
15 Retinal detachment, cystic retinoschisis.
16 Retinal haemangioma, osteoma or combined hamartoma.

Clinical types

Endophytic tumours (Fig. 17.13)
These creamy-white vascular tumours grow into the vitreous, and tumour fragments 'seed' into the vitreous cavity. They are frequently calcified.

Exophytic tumours (Fig. 17.14)
These grow into the subretinal space, causing retinal detachment. They are frequently calcified.

Diffusely infiltrating retinoblastoma
In this, the tumour infiltrates widely and may not give rise to a solid mass. It may not calcify. The onset is often later.

Tumour spread

1 Anteriorly through the ciliary body and iris, giving rise to hypopyon, iris changes.
2 Through the optic nerve to the meninges.
3 Via the anterior segment or trans-scleral spread.

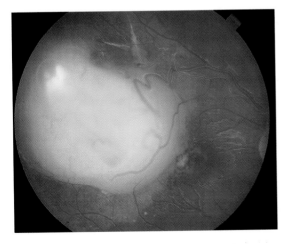

Fig. 17.12 Probable retinoma: this 5-year-old child failed a school vision test. The smooth mass was observed not to change over a period of 13 months: it showed minimal calcification on ultrasound studies.

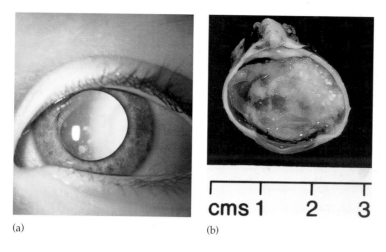

(a)

(b)

Fig. 17.13 (a) Endophytic retinoblastoma. The tumour has invaded the vitreous and seeds can be seen beyond the lens. (b) Calotte of enucleated eye with tumour filling the eye (same patient).

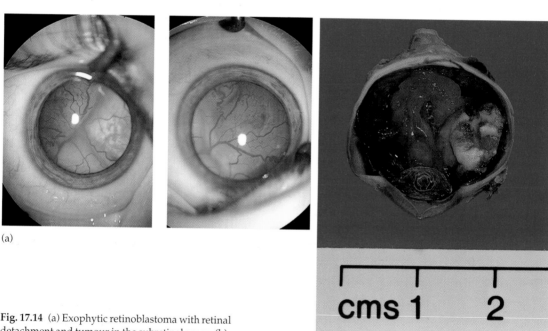

(a)

(b)

Fig. 17.14 (a) Exophytic retinoblastoma with retinal detachment and tumour in the subretinal space. (b) Calotte of enucleated eye with exophytic retinoblastoma.

4 To the orbit, then via lymphatics.
5 Haematogenous, via the choroidal circulation. Any spread outside the eye carries a poor prognosis.

Investigation
1 Ultrasound:
  (a) may show tumour formation, retinal detachment;

(b) calcium represented by high echogenicity.
2 CT scan (Fig. 17.15)—this is the best way to detect calcium.
3 Bone marrow aspiration and lumbar puncture.
4 Magnetic resonance imaging (MRI) scan—better than CT for assessment of intracranial spread.
5 Fine needle biopsy — not indicated unless the chances of the ultimate diagnosis being retinoblas-

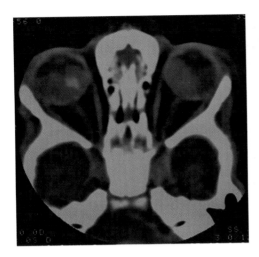

Fig. 17.15 Retinoblastoma. CT scan showing calcification within the tumour in both eyes.

toma are infinitesimally small because of the danger of trans-scleral spread.

6 Molecular genetic analysis.

7 Examination of all first-degree relatives (parents and siblings).

Treatment

The most important aspect of management is the handling of the parents. It is a shocking diagnosis that the parents have to accept quickly: detailed, sympathetic and repeated discussions are needed, together with support services for the parents at home, especially during active phases of treatment.

Enucleation

Indications
- Blind eye.
- Extensive tumour.
- Other eye unaffected or with good prognosis.
- Failure of conservative treatments.
- May need to be bilateral in advanced disease with both eyes blind.

Technique

It is important to remove as much of the optic nerve as possible. A non-metallic orbital implant may be used. Artificial eyes can be fitted as soon as 2 weeks.

Radiotherapy

External beam irradiation: indications
- Residual visual potential.
- Larger tumours.
- Tumours involving the macula or close to the optic disc.
- Multiple tumours.
- Vitreous seeding.
- Local extraocular spread.

Other local therapy

- Cryotherapy:
  (a) small anterior tumours;
  (b) especially for recurrence in already treated eyes.
- Laser therapy:
  (a) continuous wave yttrium–aluminium–garnet (YAG) or argon green;
  (b) most posterior tumours are treatable if small.

Chemotherapy

- Can produce good tumour shrinkage prior to focal therapy.
- Not helpful with vitreous seeding.
- Useful for retinoblastoma metastases but efficacy uncertain.

Patterns of regression

1 Type I — size reduction and calcified 'cottage cheese' appearance (Fig. 17.16).

2 Type II — size reduction with translucent 'fish-flesh' appearance.

Follow-up

Long-term follow-up is advisable in all cases.
- *Treated bilateral cases.* As suggested by clinical response, at increasing intervals until they are co-operative.
- *Unilateral cases* after enucleation of the affected eye:
  (a) every 3 months until 3 years old, every 6 months until 5 years old, then annually;
  (b) if molecular genetic analysis has suggested no systemic mutations, follow-up may be less frequent.

Genetic counselling mandatory for all cases; this is the province of a genetics expert and will be

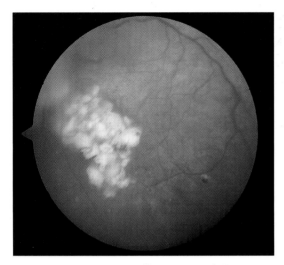

Fig. 17.16 Retinoblastoma regression following irradiation. Calcified 'cottage cheese' appearance.

greatly aided by molecular genetics, but the following are some guidelines.

1 Offspring of patients with a familial retinoblastoma have a 45% chance of developing retinoblastoma.

2 If two affected children are born to normal parents, there is a 45% chance of subsequent children developing a retinoblastoma.

3 A child with a unilateral retinoblastoma, with normal parents and no family history has a 15% chance of having a germ-line mutation and a little over 10% chance of developing a retinoblastoma in the apparently unaffected eye.

4 Offspring of children with a unilateral retinoblastoma have a less than 10% chance of developing retinoblastoma. All infants at significant risk are screened by examinations under anaesthesia.

Retinal and choroidal dystrophies

The infant with normal eyes, reduced vision and nystagmus

Leber's amaurosis
- Autosomal recessive with high intrafamilial concordance.
- Blindness from birth.
- Absent electroretinogram (ERG).

- Roving eye movements.
- Eye poking (the 'oculo-digital' sign) after infancy.
- Sluggish pupils; paradoxical pupils.
- High hypermetropia and pseudopapilloedema (Fig. 17.17).
- Normal fundi, sometimes white flecks or pigment clumping.
- Macula pigment dysplasia (Fig. 17.18).
  Later:
- thin vessels;
- pale discs.

Associated features
- Most patients are normal.
- Mental retardation.
- Renal disease.
- Cardiomyopathy.
- Deafness.

Congenital stationary night blindness (Table 17.1)
- Nystagmus — variable and not in dominant or incomplete form.
- Decreased vision, usually better than 6/60.
- Normal fundi.
- May be highly myopic.

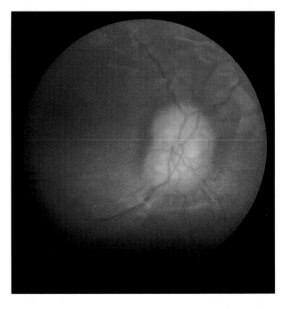

Fig. 17.17 Leber's amaurosis. High hypermetropia and pseudopapilloedema.

Table 17.1 Features of congenital stationary night blindness (CSNB).

Features	Complete CSNB	Incomplete CSNB
Dark adaptation	No rod function	Subnormal rod function
ERG rod function	No rod function	Subnormal rod function
Bright flash scotopic ERG	Negative	Negative
ERG cone responses	Normal/near normal	Normal/near normal and improve after light adaptation

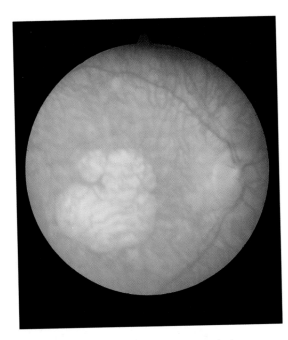

Fig. 17.18 Leber's amaurosis. Macular dysplasia.

- Paradoxical pupils (pupillary constriction in darkness).
- ERG shows normal A wave, attenuated B wave (Fig. 17.19) elevated dark adaptation thresholds.
- X-linked recessive associated with myopia.
- Autosomal recessive; lower incidence of myopia.

Prognosis
Static.

Cone dystrophy
See below.

Joubert's syndrome
- Autosomal recessive.
- Cerebellar vermis hypoplasia.
- Mild to moderate developmental delay.
- Neonatal breathing difficulties.
- Horizontal saccade palsy.
- Congenital retinal dystrophy with relatively preserved central visual function, sometimes a retinal or disc coloboma.
- ERG attenuated or absent, visual evoked potentials (VEPs) well preserved reflecting good central vision.
- It is uncertain whether or not it is progressive.
- Diagnosis:
   (a) ERG;
   (b) neuroimaging (Fig. 17.20).

Peroxisomal diseases
Peroxisomes catabolise very long chain fatty acids, pipecolic acid and phytanic acid. They are involved in the synthesis of phospholipids.

Zellweger's syndrome (cerebro-hepato-renal syndrome)
- Autosomal recessive.
- Dysmorphic; bulging forehead, micrognathia.
- Hepatomegaly.
- Renal cysts.
- Hypotonia.
- Regression and seizures.
  Eye features:
- nystagmus;
- corneal clouding;
- cataract;
- retinal dystrophy with severely subnormal ERG.

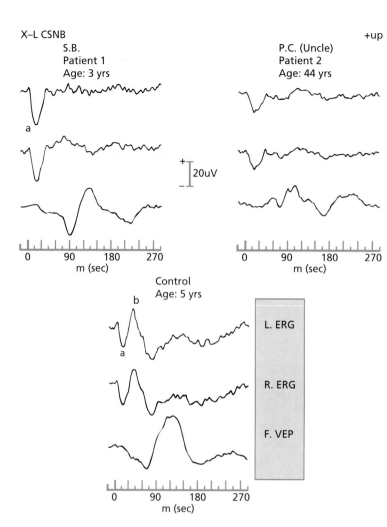

X–L CSNB

S.B.
Patient 1
Age: 3 yrs

a

+up

P.C. (Uncle)
Patient 2
Age: 44 yrs

+
20uV
–

0   90   180   270
m (sec)

0   90   180   270
m (sec)

Control
Age: 5 yrs

b

a

L. ERG

R. ERG

F. VEP

0   90   180   270
m (sec)

Fig. 17.19 Mixed cone/rod ERGs and visual evoked potentials from a 3-year-old boy and his maternal uncle, both of whom have X-linked congenital stationary night blindness (upper traces), the appearance of a 5-year-old control (lower traces). Note both patients have a negative ERG with a clearly discernible A wave.

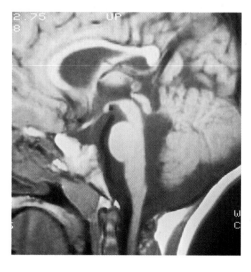

Fig. 17.20 Joubert's syndrome. MRI scan showing cerebellar vermis hypoplasia and a large fourth ventricle.

Neonatal adrenoleucodystrophy
- Autosomal recessive.
- Developmental regression and deafness.
- Uncontrollable seizures; hypotonia.
- Optic atrophy.
- Retinal dystrophy.
- The ERG is subnormal and deteriorates.
- Early death.

Infantile Refsum's disease
(infantile phytanic acid storage disease)
Similar to neonatal adrenoleucodsytrophy with later onset and longer lifespan.

Diagnosis of peroxisomal diseases
Abnormal serum levels of very long chain fatty acids, pipecolic acids, phytanic acid and bile acids.

Alström's disease
- Autosomal recessive.
- Diabetes mellitus.
- Obesity, skin changes (acanthosis nigricans).
- Deafness in second decade.
- Early onset retinal dystrophy with reduced ERG.

Jeune's syndrome
- Autosomal recessive.
- Congenital asphyxiating thoracic dystrophy.
- Polydactyly and other skeletal abnormalities.
- ERG shows subnormal rod and cone responses.

Osteopetrosis
Apart from the bone changes, sometimes these patients have abnormal ERGs.

Others
1 Cohen's syndrome:
   (a) autosomal recessive;
   (b) short stature;
   (c) microcephaly;
   (d) mental retardation;
   (e) dysmorphism.
2 Senior's syndrome:
   (a) autosomal recessive;
   (b) juvenile nephronophthisis (medullary cystic renal disease);

(c) retinal dystrophy of later onset or with nystagmus.
3 Methylmalonic and other acidurias.

The infant with normal eyes, nystagmus and photophobia

Rod monochromatism (achromatopsia)
- Autosomal recessive.
- Complete colour blindness.
- Nystagmus (often high frequency, low amplitude).
- Photophobia from infancy.
- Good night vision.
- Reduced acuity.
- Sluggish pupil reactions and paradoxical pupils (pupillary constriction in the dark).
- High hypermetropia.
- Asymmetrical monocular optokinetic nystagmus (OKN).
- ERG shows abnormal scotopic responses and flicker, with normal scotopic responses, reduced VEPs (Fig. 17.21).

Dyschromatopsia
- Similar to achromatopsia but probably affects the cone system only, i.e. red or green cones only.
- VEPs present.

Blue cone monochromatism
- X-linked recessive.
- Normal rods and blue cones.
- ERGs show very small A and B wave amplitude.
- Mostly diagnosed by psychophysics.
- Myopia, mild photophobia, nystagmus and reduced acuity.

Leber's amaurosis
Some patients are significantly photophobic (see above).

Maculopathies
Occasionally patients with Stargardt's disease or other maculopathies are photophobic in infancy.

Others
1 *Alström's disease*. Patients may be photophobic and have cone defects initially.

Rod monochromatism (SI)

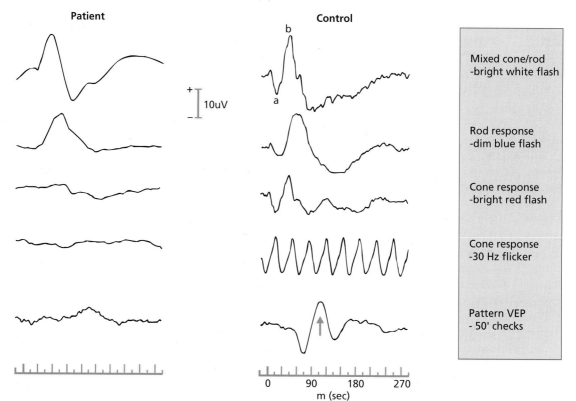

Patient   Control

10uV

Mixed cone/rod
-bright white flash

Rod response
-dim blue flash

Cone response
-bright red flash

Cone response
-30 Hz flicker

Pattern VEP
- 50' checks

0   90   180   270
m (sec)

Fig. 17.21 Flash ERGs and VEPs from a young patient with rod monochromatism (left side) and a control subject (right side). She produces well-preserved rod-mediated ERGs to bright and dim white flashes but no discernible cone-mediated ERGs to red flashes at 3 per second or 30 per second flicker. Her Pattern VEPs to 50′ checks (and larger check sizes) were broad and delayed.

2 *Cystinosis.* Some patients with cystinosis who are photophobic have a retinal dystrophy.
3 *Cone–rod dystrophies.* These patients present with signs and symptoms of cone dystrophy but later develop clinical and neurophysiological signs of rod involvement, including night blindness.

Other conditions
Albinism and aniridia.

Children with mainly macular changes, colour vision and visual acuity defects
Progressive cone dystrophy
• Autosomal recessive or autosomal dominant.
• Onset after infancy, up to early adulthood.
• Photophobia.
• Nystagmus sometimes develops.
• Bull's eye maculopathy (Fig. 17.22).
• ERG: normal rod responses, absent or reduced cone responses.
• VEP reduced.
• Acuity of central field and colour vision reduced.

Stargardt's disease: fundus flavimaculatus
• Autosomal recessive.
• Present with insidious acuity loss.
• Bilateral, symmetrical.
• Fluorescein angiography shows window defects

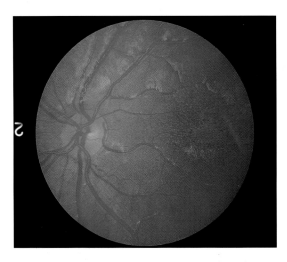

Fig. 17.22 Progressive cone dystrophy with bull's eye maculopathy.

Box 17.4 Bull's eye maculopathies

1 (Progressive) cone dystrophy.
2 Stargardt's disease.
3 Batten's disease.
4 Cone–rod dystrophies.
5 Drug toxicity.
6 Others:
  (a) Hallervorden–Spatz disease;
  (b) mucolipidosis type IV;
  (c) fucosidosis;
  (d) Bardet–Biedl syndrome;
  (e) benign concentric macular dystrophy;
  (f) fenestrated sheen dystrophy.

---

due to retinal pigment epithelial (RPE) changes and 'dark' choroid (Fig. 17.23).

• Funduscopy shows macular pigment disturbance.

• 'Fish-tail' flavimaculatus lesions, mostly in midperiphery.

• Progression — acuity reduced to 6/60–3/60 with mostly full peripheral fields.

• Normal ERG and EOG in early disease, VEP abnormal early.

• Gene locus at 1p21–p13.

Best's vitelliform dystrophy

• Autosomal dominant.

• Variable expression, all first-degree relatives must be examined.

• Early onset.

• Bilateral, asymmetrical.

• EOG subnormal, ERG, dark adaptation and fields normal.

• Classical vitelliform lesions (Fig. 17.24).

• Disrupted vitelliform lesions (Fig. 17.25).

• Subretinal scarring.

• Visual acuity between 6/6 and 6/60, prognosis reasonably good.

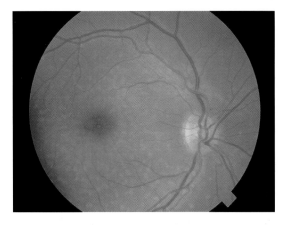

Fig. 17.23 Fundus flavimaculatus—'fish-tail' lesions and a mild maculopathy.

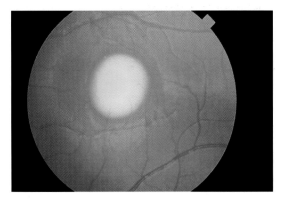

Fig. 17.24 Best's disease. Classical vitelliform lesion resembling an egg yolk 'sunny-side-up'.

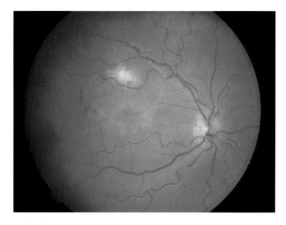

Fig. 17.25 Ruptured vitelliform lesion which has partially dispersed leaving a subretinal scar.

• Fluorescein angiography shows macular hyperfluorescence. Vitelliform lesions block choroidal hyperfluorescence.

Pattern dystrophies
• Variable inheritance.
• Onset usually in late childhood or adolescence.
• Moderately reduced acuity.
• ERG normal, EOG may be mildly abnormal.
• Macula shows pigmentation in a 'butterfly' or reticular form (Fig. 17.26).

Other macular dystrophies
• *Bifocal macular dystrophy*:
  (a) retinal atrophy nasal and temporal to the optic disc;
  (b) autosomal dominant.
• *North Carolina macular dystrophy*:
  (a) autosomal dominant;
  (b) possibly stationary;
  (c) very variable, acuities normal, or as low as 3/60;
  (d) central, retinal and choroidal atrophy;
  (e) EOG and ERG normal.
• *Fenestrated sheen macular dystrophy and dominant cystoid macular oedema* — see D. Taylor (ed.), Chapter 45, *Paediatric Ophthalmology*, 2nd edn, 1997, Blackwell Science, Oxford.

Systemic disease with predominantly macular onset of retinal disease
• *Batten's disease*. Juvenile Batten's disease usually presents as a macular dystrophy, often with a bull's eye appearance (see Chapter 20).
• *Hallervorden–Spatz disease* (see below).

Macular 'coloboma' and dysplasia
These are variable defects in the retinal pigment epithelium and choroid, sometimes with an ectatic area at the posterior pole. Visual acuity, colour vision loss, ERG and VEP abnormalities depend on the extent of the coloboma.

Macular dysplasia is seen in some retinal dystrophies including Leber's amaurosis and retinitis pigmentosa. It appears as RPE atrophy, sometimes with underlying choroidal defects.

Foveal retinoschisis
See Juvenile X-linked retinoschisis, Chapter 16.

Foveal hypoplasia
This is detected by the finding of reduced acuity, contrast sensitivity and colour vision and a loss of the macular profiles seen, particularly on indirect ophthalmoscopy or slit lamp biomicroscopy. Central foveal reflexes are absent and the macular hill may be defective. It occurs commonly in:
1 albinism;
2 aniridia;
3 achromatopsia;

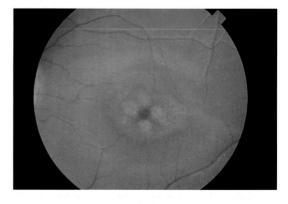

Fig. 17.26 Pattern dystrophy.

4 may be isolated, accounting for poor acuity, but albinism must be excluded in these patients.

Children with apparently acquired night vision defects or mainly and initially peripheral visual loss

Stationary conditions

These are congenital conditions, but often present as though they are acquired.

1 Congenital stationary night blindness (see above).

2 Oguchi's disease:

(a) autosomal recessive;

(b) mostly Japanese;

(c) present in childhood with night blindness;

(d) negative ERG;

(e) yellow phosphorescent fundus coloration, becoming normal after several hours dark adaptation (Mizuo phenomenon).

3 Aland Island eye disease:

(a) iris transillumination, pale fundi, foveal hypoplasia;

(b) night blindness;

(c) negative ERG, VEPs do not show albino-type misrouting.

4 Fundus albipunctatus:

(a) autosomal recessive, congenital night blindness;

(b) multiple discrete elevated white dots in the RPE;

(c) EOG and ERG abnormal in the light-adapted eye.

5 Oregon eye disease—see D. Taylor (ed.), Chapter 44, *Paediatric Ophthalmology*, 2nd edn, 1997, Blackwell Science, Oxford.

Progressive retinal and choroidal dystrophies

Retinitis pigmentosa

A group of progressive retinal degenerations with a similar phenotype but with different rates of progression and severity and different modes of inheritance.

Incidence. Approximately 1 in 4000.

Symptoms. The following symptoms are common.

• Night blindness.

• Reduced peripheral vision; occasionally a ring scotoma.

• Reduced or absent rod and cone ERGs.

• Acuity and colour vision preserved until late in the progress of the disease.

Fundus changes. The following fundus changes are common.

• Retinal vascular narrowing (Fig. 17.27)—subtle in early cases, marked later.

• RPE changes:

(a) widespread, peripheral at first;

(b) macular sparing;

(c) progressive;

(d) pigment clumping;

(e) bone spicules (Fig. 17.28) most frequent.

• Macular changes:

(a) pigmentation;

(b) epiretinal membranes;

(c) cystoid macular oedema.

• Myopia frequent.

• Cataracts occur as retinal changes advance.

• Vitreous detaches early.

• Optic nerve atrophy and drusen in advanced cases.

Anatomical subtypes—

• Diffuse.

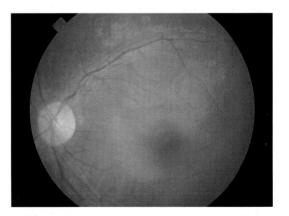

Fig. 17.27 Retinitis pigmentosa in a 6 year old. The only symptom was night blindness. Peripheral pigment clumping is present and the arterioles are narrow. There are minimal posterior polar changes.

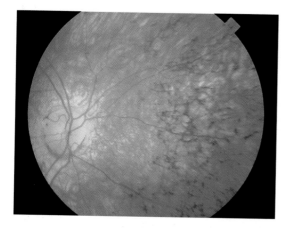

Fig. 17.28 Retinitis pigmentosa. 'Bone spicule' formation in the midperiphery and arteriolar narrowing.

- Peripheral.
- Macular sparing.
- Early macular involvement:
  (a) sectoral;
  (b) unilateral (probably highly asymmetrical).

Genetic subtypes—
- Autosomal dominant:
  (a) incomplete penetrance.;
  (b) later onset of symptoms;
  (c) more slow progression, sometimes good acuity preserved for many decades;
  (d) rhodopsin gene (chromosome 3) and peripherin/RDS (chromosome 6) mutations.
- Autosomal recessive:
  (a) parent consanguinity frequent in some countries;
  (b) parents normal;
  (c) early onset, relatively rapid progression to blindness by the second or third decade.
- X-linked recessive:
  (a) males only affected—no direct male-to-male transmission;
  (b) early onset, rapid progression similar to autosomal recessive form;
  (c) gene loci Xp11 andXp21.

Differential diagnoses. The most important differential diagnoses are with treatable forms of phenocopies such as avitaminosis A, abetalipoprotinaemia and acquired vitamin A and E deficiency as in malabsorption syndromes. Refsum's disease may have a similar retinal pigmentary retinopathy.

Traumatic pigmented retinopathy is usually unilateral.

Treatment of retinitis pigmentosa—
- Cataracts may warrant surgery.
- Macular oedema may be improved by the use of acetazolamide. No other effective treatments have been proven.

Molecular genetics of retinitis pigmentosa. For details of the molecular genetics of retinitis pigmentosa see D. Taylor (ed), Chapters 44 & 45, *Paediatric Ophthalmology,* 2nd edn, 1997, Blackwell Science, Oxford.

Choroideraemia
- X-linked recessive.
- Night blindness.
- Peripheral visual loss.
- Late central visual loss.
- Carriers have mottled retinal pigment abnormalities.
- Affected boys have equatorial pigment epithelial and choriocapillaris atrophy with scalloped edges (Fig. 17.29).
- Gradual progression over decades.
- ERG extinguished early.
- Xp22.1–q21.31.

Gyrate atrophy
- Autosomal recessive—chromosome 10.
- Night vision defects in early childhood.
- Peripheral visual field constriction.
- Progressive.
- Myopia.
- Raised plasma ornithine.
- Midperipheral 'punched out' chorioretinal atrophy (Fig. 17.30).
- Some patients respond to pyridoxine or prolene supplementation.
- ERG — abnormal; scotopic early, latent extinguished.

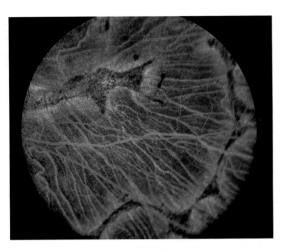

Fig. 17.29 Choroideraemia—fluorescein angiogram showing characteristic scalloped appearance given by the surviving RPE and loss of choriocapillaris.

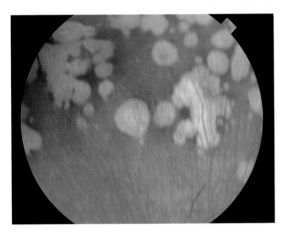

Fig. 17.30 Gyrate atrophy with hyperornithinaemia. This 9-year-old girl presented with night blindness. Although the posterior pole was normal the mid and far periphery show the typical atrophic areas.

Mitochondrial cytopathies
- Lactic acidosis.
- Myopathies, especially facial.
- Deafness.
- Cardiac conduction defects (Kearns–Sayre syndrome).
- Progressive retinal dystrophy with abnormal ERG.

Biedl–Bardet syndrome
- Autosomal recessive, gene at 11q221 or 16q13–q22.
- Obesity.
- Mental dullness or retardation.
- Post-axial polydactyly.
- Hypogenitalism.
- Renal dystrophy.
- Progressive retinal dystrophy:
  (a) variable progression, onset usually by 5 years;
  (b) bull's eye occasionally seen;
  (c) arteriolar narrowing and optic disc pallor;
  (d) peripheral pigmentation only late (Fig. 17.31).
- The Laurence–Moon syndrome is similar, without obesity or polydactyly.

Hallervorden–Spatz syndrome
- Progressive extrapyramidal disease.
- Dementia.
- Retinal dystrophy.
- ERG non-recordable.

Juvenile Batten's disease
(See Chapter 20.) Juvenile Batten's disease usually has night vision defects at a later stage.

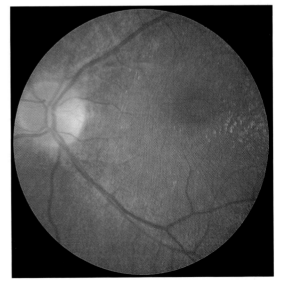

Fig. 17.31 Biedl–Bardet syndrome. Retinal dystrophy with retinal oedema.

Cockayne's syndrome
- Deafness.
- Dwarfism.
- Progeria.
- Mental regression.
- Progressive retinal dystrophy.
- ERG extinguished early.

Mucopolysaccharidoses and mucolipidoses
See Chapter 20.

Acquired peripheral visual defects
- Avitaminosis A and E.
- Desferrioxamine toxicity.
- Refsum's disease.
- Trauma, usually unilateral.

Box 17.5 Eye abnormalities and deafness

1 Usher's syndrome (autosomal recessive).
Usher's type I:
  (a) profound congenital deafness;
  (b) vestibular dysfunction;
  (c) retinal dystrophy with early acuity defect;
  (d) genes at 14q and 11q.
Usher's type II:
  (a) retinal dystrophy with later acuity defect;
  (b) high-frequency deafness;
  (c) intact vestibular reflexes;
  (d) gene locus 1q14.
2 Cockaynes' syndrome.
3 Alstrom's syndrome.
4 Refsum's disease.
5 Mitochondrial cytopathy.
6 Peroxisomal disorders.
7 Mucopolysaccharidoses.
8 Flynn–Aird syndrome:
  (a) autosomal dominant;
  (b) retinal dystrophy, cataract, myopia;
  (c) deafness, ataxia, skin atrophy, baldness;
  (d) peripheral neuritis, ataxia, dementia.
9 Choroideraemia–deafness syndrome.
10 Meningitis.
11 Norrie's disease.
12 CHARGE association.
13 Bone disease, osteopetrosis, craniometaphyseal dysplasia.
14 Stickler's syndrome.
15 Duanes and Möbius syndromes.
16 Neurofibromatosis types 1 and 2.

Pigmented paravenous atrophy
- Night blindness.
- Paravenous pigmentation and atrophy.
- Progression uncertain.

Flecked retinas

1 Fundus flavimaculatus — see Stargardt's disease, pp. 144–145.
2 Fundus albipunctatus—see above.
3 Dominant drusen:
  (a) autosomal dominant;
  (b) very variable expression;
  (c) posterior polar white/yellow drusen;
  (d) rarely symptomatic in childhood.
4 Others.
  (a) *Bietti's dystrophy*:
    (i) autosomal recessive;
    (ii) retinal and corneal crystals.
  (b) *Kandori's dystrophy*—stationary midperipheral yellow flecks.
  (c) *Retinitis pigmentosa*:
    (i) some cases have yellow-appearing flecks in the midperiphery;
    (ii) then it is sometimes known as retinitis punctata albescens.
  (d) *Alport's syndrome*.

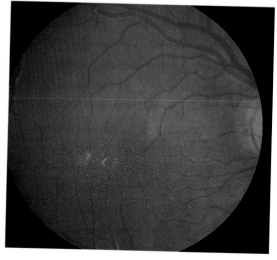

Fig. 17.32 Sjögren–Larsson syndrome showing macular crystal formation.

(e) *Sjögren–Larsson syndrome*:
   (i) autosomal recessive;
   (ii) spastic diplegia;
   (iii) mental retardation;
   (iv) ichthyosis;

   (v) macular crystals (Fig. 17.32).
(f) *Avitaminosis A.*
(g) Others—see D. Taylor (ed.), Chapter 48, *Paediatric Ophthalmology*, 2nd edn, 1997, Blackwell Science, Oxford.

18: Anterior Visual Pathway Defects

Optic nerve: developmental anomalies

The optic nerve is 75% of adult size by birth and 95% by 1 year of age. The optic disc appears somewhat pale when compared to an adult's, it is normally myelinated at birth and the physiological cup, although present in some cases, is very small.

The grey disc

This is a grey appearance of the optic disc seen in early infancy associated with poor vision and thought to be a form of delayed visual maturation (see Chapter 2).

Optic disc pigmentation

1 Congenital anomalies (Fig. 18.1).
2 Post-inflammatory pigmentation (Fig. 18.2).
3 Melanocytoma. This is a jet-black benign tumour.
4 Aicardi's syndrome (Fig. 18.3). This syndrome occurs in girls with infantile spasms, severe retardation, ectopic cerebral grey matter, absence of the corpus collusum, vertebral anomalies and characteristic lacunar defects in the retina and colobomas.
5 Retinal pigment epithelial hamartoma. This may involve the optic discs and be pigmented. They are vascular on fluorescein angiography with radiating folds into the surrounding retina. They have been noted particularly with neurofibromatosis type 2 but may occur as an isolated lesion (see Chapter 17).
6 Pigmented anomalous discs. Colobomatous and dysplastic discs may also be pigmented.

Congenital vascular abnormalities of the optic disc

1 Cilioretinal arteries:
  (a) may be multiple;
  (b) arise from the ciliary circulation;
  (c) usually small but occasionally large;

  (d) may occur in 50% of the population (Fig. 18.4).
2 Opticociliary veins:
  (a) veins connecting the intraocular venous system via choroidal veins to vortex veins;
  (b) high myopia;
  (c) chronic obstruction of the central retinal vein, i.e. in glioma and meningioma (Fig. 18.4).

Situs inversus

Tilted optic discs which occur usually in high myopes with the appearance of the disc being in the 'wrong' direction, i.e. the vessels tend to loop nasally rather than temporally.

Haemangiomas of the optic disc

Haemangiomas usually involve the optic disc and peripapillary retina and may be a manifestation of von Hippel–Lindau syndrome (see Chapters 17 and 24).

Bergmeister's papilla and prepapillary vascular loops

Bergmeister's papillas represent remnants of the hyaloid vessels and they appear as small whitish grey elevations in front of the optic disc (Fig. 18.5).

Prepapillary vascular loops are not uncommon. Sometimes they are marked and tortuous (Fig. 18.6) or corkscrew in shape, projecting anteriorly from the optic disc. They may obstruct in adult life.

Myelinated nerve fibres

In 1% of the population, myelin extends anterior to the cribriform plate. Myelinated nerve fibres are usually contiguous with the optic disc but occasionally separate from it. There is a field defect related to the area of myelination (Fig. 18.7).

There is an association between unilateral widespread myelinated nerve fibres, high myopia and amblyopia.

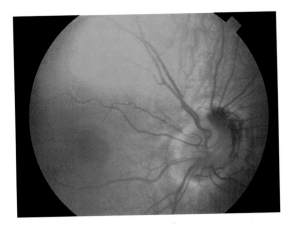

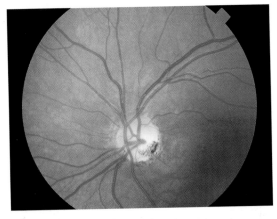

Fig. 18.1 Congenital optic disc pigmentation. Linear pigmentation concentric with the optic disc margin.

Fig. 18.2 Optic disc pigmentation following optic neuritis.

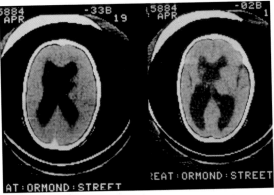

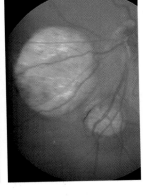

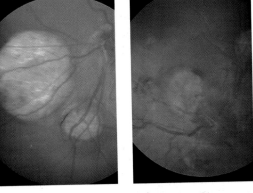

Fig. 18.3 Aicardi's syndrome. Punched-out chorioretinal lesions with dysplasic optic discs. The chorioretinal lesions consist of clear-cut defects in the retinal pigment epithelium with the neural retina overlying it intact and the underlying choroid being abnormal, allowing sclera to show through. The CT scan shows subependymal heterotopia in a girl with seizures.

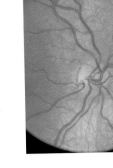

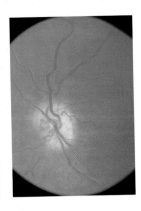

Fig. 18.4 This patient has a chiasmal and left optic nerve glioma. The left eye shows optic atrophy and opticociliary shunt vessels. The right eye shows a single cilioretinal artery in the inferotemporal quadrant. This is a common congenital anomaly.

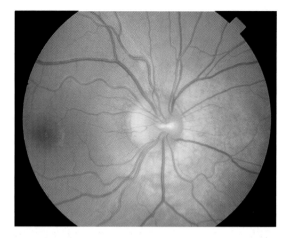

Fig. 18.5 Bergmeister's papilla showing a more or less solid glial elevation anterior to the optic disc.

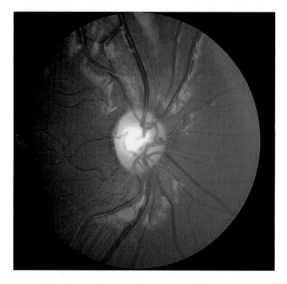

Fig. 18.6 Corkscrew prepapillary vascular loop.

Drusen

Drusen appears as a swollen optic disc with, eventually, a lumpy outline. Sometimes, especially in older children, crystalline drusen bodies can be seen in the disc (Fig. 18.8). The capillaries are not dilated and do not usually leak fluorescein. The drusen may autofluoresce (i.e. fluoresce before the injection of fluorescein). There may be vascular anomalies including trifurcation and anomalous vessels.

Haemorrhages adjacent to the disc are not uncommon.

It may be a progressive condition. It is associated with retinitis pigmentosa, hypotelorism and mandibulofacial dysostosis.

It may be detected by computerized tomography (CT) scanning or ultrasound.

Papilloedema in children

Papilloedema is the appearance of the optic disc associated with raised intracranial pressure. The characteristic appearance is:

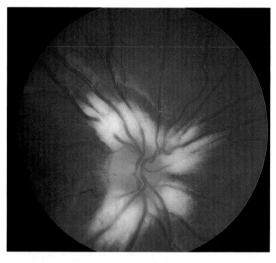

Fig. 18.7 Myelinated nerve fibres adjacent to the optic disc.

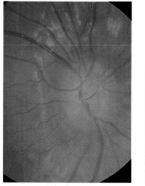 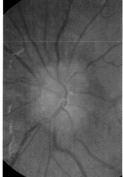

Fig. 18.8 Optic nerve drusen giving pseudopapilloedema in a 10-year-old child with headaches: note the anomalous blood vessels and the lumpy crystalline drusen bodies.

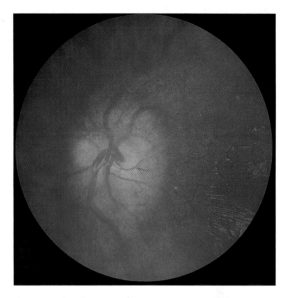

Fig. 18.9 Papilloedema in a patient with neurofibromatosis and a chiasmal glioma. The swelling of the optic disc with dilated veins, haemorrhages, a few exudates and dilated capillaries is most marked in the upper and lower poles. The eye has a temporal hemianopia and the fibres that are swollen are those subserving the intact nasal fields. The horizontal band of relative lack of swelling is in the area of the disc that is atrophic from loss of nerve fibres. The superior poles, although also atrophic, are covered by the fibres from the intact nasal field and are therefore swollen.

> **Box 18.1 Pseudopapilloedema**
>
> **1** Myelinated nerve fibres.
> **2** Drusen.
> **3** Hypermetropia.
> **4** Myopia.
> **5** Disc infiltration.
> **6** Tilted disc.

- congested neurones seen especially adjacent to the optic disc;
- the disc is elevated;
- the peripapillary capillaries are dilated;
- swelling of the nerve fibres and oedema extends into the retina giving circumferential choroidal folds;
- the blind spot is enlarged and, if nerve fibre loss occurs, nerve fibre bundle defects occur on visual field studies;
- venous pulsation, if present, suggests that the intracranial pressure is normal;
- haemorrhages, in particular splinter haemorrhages, nerve fibre infarcts and macular star formation occur with more severe papilloedema (Figs 18.9 & 18.10).

Symptoms of papilloedema

Papilloedema itself is asymptomatic unless there is vascular or neuronal compromise; there may also be symptoms from the intracranial disease.

1 Obscurations. These are posture-related, seconds-long asymmetrical, blackouts or greyouts, particularly on standing and in severe hydrocephalus.

2 Visual distortion due to retinal oedema, colour vision loss.

3 Blind spot enlargement may be symptomatic.

Management

Clinical evaluation including acuity, colour vision, fields and visual evoked potentials (VEPs), and neurological assessment. It is important to evaluate carefully the visual and headache symptoms for evidence of change, and to see how much the child is affected by them.

The management of the raised intracranial pressure usually consists of neuroimaging to detect

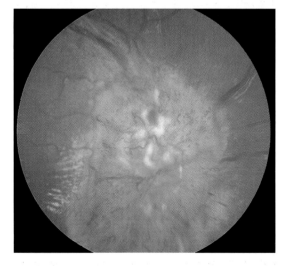

Fig. 18.10 Severe papilloedema with gross elevation, haemorrhages, exudates, macular star, dilated veins and cotton wool spots on the optic disc.

any underlying abnormalities (tumours, meningeal infiltration, meningitis, etc.), measuring the intracranial pressure by lumbar puncture or by a transcranial transducer.

Benign intracranial hypertension

Patients who have normal neuroimaging and no other neurological signs have 'benign intracranial hypertension' or 'pseudotumour cerebri'. This tends to occur in obese females but often occurs in other groups, sometimes after treatment with steroids (especially when too rapidly withdrawn), vitamin A, antibiotics, oral contraceptives and with lead toxicity. Treatment is indicated if the symptoms are severe, or if the optic disc is severely swollen, with any evidence of an optic neuropathy. Any underlying cause, such as drug use, is eliminated, or if the problem has been brought about by too rapid reduction of steroids, a higher dose is used and withdrawn more slowly. Acetazolamide may reduce the headache, but the effect often does not last long, and the side-effects may not be justified in the longer term.

Optic nerve sheath fenestration may be considered for patients who have marked and increasing obscurations. Ventriculoperitoneal or ventriculo-atrial shunting may be indicated if conservative measures fail.

Optic nerve aplasia

This is very rare, usually associated with widespread ocular abnormalities. It is usually unilateral, occasionally bilateral. The eyes are usually blind and there is no optic disc or vessels and there may be retinal abnormalities.

Optic nerve hypoplasia

Bilateral severe optic nerve hypoplasia presents as blindness in infancy. Lesser degrees may cause minor visual defects and present at any time in childhood, either as a failed school test, strabismus or nystagmus. Unilateral optic nerve hypoplasia presents as strabismus with a relative afferent pupil defect and unsteady fixation in the affected eye. See-saw nystagmus may occur (Figs 18.11 & 18.12).

> **Box 18.2 The swollen optic disc in childhood**
>
> *Bilateral*
> 1 Papilloedema (raised intracranial pressure):
>   (a) hydrocephalus;
>   (b) benign intracranial hypertension.
> 2 Hypertension.
> 3 Papillitis (optic neuritis).
> 4 Bilateral cases of unilateral causes.
>
> *Unilateral*
> 1 Pseudopapilloedema:
>   (a) drusen;
>   (b) myelinated nerve fibres;
>   (c) hypermetropia;
>   (d) myopia;
>   (e) glial anomalies.
> 2 Tumours:
>   (a) haemangioma;
>   (b) mulberry tumour of tuberous sclerosis;
>   (c) retinal hamartoma;
>   (d) retinoblastoma;
>   (e) optic nerve glioma;
>   (f) leukaemia.
> 3 Uveitis.
> 4 Ischaemic optic neuropathy.
> 5 Papillitis.
> 6 Chronic hypotony.
> 7 Papilloedema (papilloedema may be very asymmetrical due to anomalous nerves).

Amblyopia may be superadded to the organic defect and must be treated, as must refractive errors.

The ophthalmoscopic appearance is of a small disc with sometimes a ring surrounding it, which represents sclera, bared by a hole in the retinal pigment epithelium.

A tilted optic disc may represent minor degrees of segmental optic nerve hypoplasia. There may be an association with developmental tumours of the anterior visual system.

Vision in optic nerve hypoplasia

Vision is variably reduced in optic nerve hypoplasia, related to the number of neurones that have failed to develop. Acuity can be normal or the patient can be completely blind. It is very difficult to determine the level of vision in a small baby with partial optic nerve hypoplasia, so prognosis should be very guarded to avoid being over- or underopti-

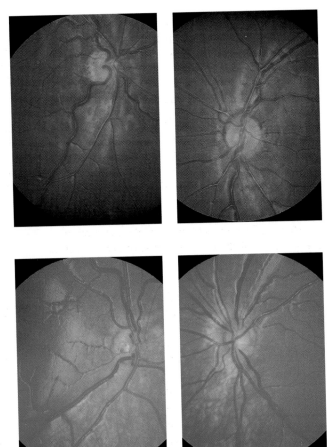

Fig. 18.11 Unilateral optic nerve hypoplasia. Although unilateral, even if there is no CT abnormality, these children must be followed throughout their childhood for growth defects.

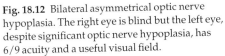

Fig. 18.12 Bilateral asymmetrical optic nerve hypoplasia. The right eye is blind but the left eye, despite significant optic nerve hypoplasia, has 6/9 acuity and a useful visual field.

mistic. Temporal visual field defects are common. The VEPs are reduced. The electroretinogram (ERG) may be enhanced due to deafferentation. Colour vision is reduced in proportion to the acuity defects. Nystagmus may be present, sometimes see-saw.

Genetics and aetiology

Optic nerve hypoplasia is not familial (except when it occurs in association with aniridia) and the recurrence risk is low.

Environmental causes

- Drugs taken during pregnancy:
  (a) antiepileptic drugs;
  (b) alcohol;
  (c) cocaine;
  (d) LSD.
- Maternal diabetes.

Associations

Aniridia, central nervous system defects including hydranencephaly, anencephaly, porencephaly, many midline defects, in particular holoprosencephaly. In septo-optic dysplasia there is an absence of the septum pellucidum or more widespread brain malformations up to holoprosencephaly, optic nerve hypoplasia and a variety of hormonal defects, both anterior and posterior pituitary.

Management

1 Infants who present as a result of optic nerve hypoplasia usually have poor vision and nystagmus

and warrant visual assessment clinically and neuro-physiologically and a magnetic resonance imaging (MRI) scan.

2 Older children being found to have optic nerve hypoplasia do not necessarily have to be scanned if they are perfectly normal in development and growth.

3 Growth should be monitored throughout childhood.

4 Newborn babies' parents should be warned about taking them to hot climates in which they may be dehydrated if they have a posterior pituitary defect.

5 Associated developmental abnormalities related to brain defects must be looked for clinically or by neuroimaging in patients presenting in early infancy, or if there is any hint of developmental delay.

6 Associated amblyopia must be treated.

7 Early attention must be paid to visual rehabilitation, stimulation and education (see Chapter 2).

Optic disc anomalies with midline defects

Midline facial clefts, meningocoeles and ence-phalocoeles may be associated with not only brain defects but also optic nerve abnormalities (Fig. 18.13). The facial clefts may be minimal and the optic discs are usually dysplastic rather than typically colobomatous.

Optic disc coloboma

Colobomas of the optic disc are caused by defective closure of the fetal fissure and usually affect the inferior part of the retina and choroid. Some colobomas are atypical and do not extend inferiorly. They may be associated with colobomas of the choroid, ciliary body or iris.

Visual effects

These depend on how much the macular and retina are involved and whether there is an associated refractive error or amblyopia.

Assessment of the infant's vision is by clinical means and by VEPs and ERGs.

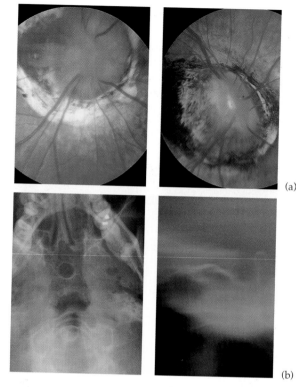

(a)

(b)

Fig. 18.13 (a) The optic discs of this child, who presented with a squint and growth defect, are dysplastic. (b) The radiological studies show that there is a defect in the floor of the pituitary fossa associated with a midline meningocoele.

Warburg's classification (modified)
1 Typical:
  (a) iris coloboma
    (i) complete (keyhole)
    (ii) peripheral
    (iii) notch in the pupil
    (iv) pigment epithelium defect (heterochromia of the iris);
  (b) coloboma of the ciliary body;
  (c) coloboma of the choroid
    (i) partial
    (ii) complete;
  (d) coloboma of the optic nerve
    (i) typical, may be associated with cyst
    (ii) 'special', e.g. pits, Pedler's coloboma, morning glory abnormality.

2 Atypical (coloboma outside the fetal fissure).
3 Macular coloboma.

Typical optic disc colobomas (Figs 18.14 & 18.15) are usually associated with an inferonasal chorio-retinal defect. They may be hugely excavated or just be associated with subtle changes in the retinal pigment epithelium (Fig. 18.16).

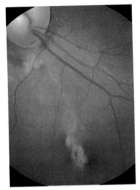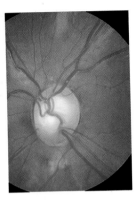

Fig. 18.16 The slightly anomalous optic nerves in this child with the CHARGE association (see p. 160) is associated with a mild chorioretinal defect inferiorly indicating the basic colobomatous nature of the defect.

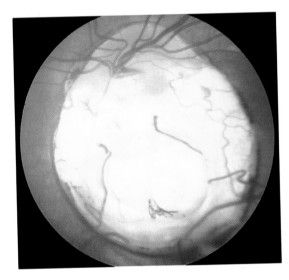

Fig. 18.14 Typical large optic nerve coloboma.

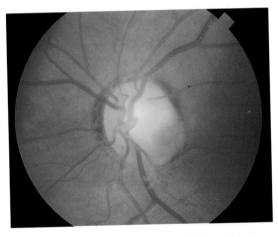

Fig. 18.17 Optic disc pit. Left eye showing temporal optic disc pit. Left eye showing temporal optic disc pit associated with cystoid macular oedema.

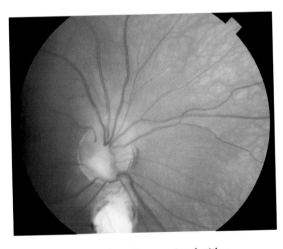

Fig. 18.15 An anomalous disc associated with a chorioretinal coloboma in a child with the CHARGE association with preserved central visual functions.

Optic disc pits

These are probably related to colobomas and usually occur on the temporal margin (Fig. 18.17). Over 50% of patients will develop serous retinopathy with visual symptoms, which may be complicated with subretinal neovascularisation. Treatment by laser and internal gas tamponade may be the treatment of choice for those patients who have acuity loss that is progressive and which does not improve with time.

Intraocular abnormalities with colobomas
- Preserved hyaloid vascular system.
- Lens notches.
- Cataract.
- Dysplastic retina around the optic disc which may include:
  (a) lacrimal tissue;
  (b) cartilage with ossification;
  (c) adipose and smooth muscle tissue.

Ocular complications of colobomas
- Retinal detachment.
- Subretinal neovascularization.
- Disciform degeneration.
- Glaucoma from associated anterior segment malformation.

Pedler's coloboma
These are usually uniocular, excavated discs with thickened (overlaid) peripapillary retina probably containing a wide variety of non-ocular tissue. Sometimes contraction has been observed (Fig. 18.18).

Peripapillary staphyloma
The sclera around the optic disc is ectatic and relatively myopic and usually appears pale.

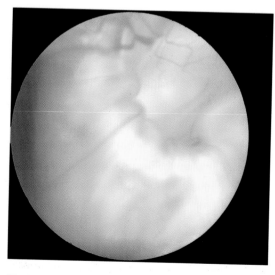

Fig. 18.18 Pedler's coloboma. A coloboma of the optic disc with overlay of the peripapillary retina.

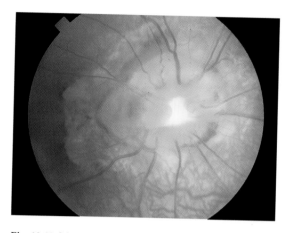

Fig. 18.19 Morning glory anomaly. There is a glial anomaly with a persistent hyaloid system and the retinal vessels radiate from around the optic disc. At birth, the peripapillary retina was detached: it settled spontaneously.

Morning glory anomaly
This is usually unilateral with an elevated area in front of the disc around which there is sometimes pigment clumping. The blood vessels exit the optic disc radially. There is usually a glial tuft passing anteriorly to a hyaloid system of vessel. The vision is poor. It is probably non-genetic (Fig. 18.19).

Systemic associations of colobomas
Chromosomal syndromes
- Trisomy 13.
- Cat eye syndrome (tri- or tetrasomy 22pter).
- 4P syndrome (Wolf–Hirschorn syndrome).
- Triploidy.
- Others.

Systemic anomalies due to a single gene defect
CHARGE association
- Choanal atresia.
- Conotruncal and heart defects.
- Ear abnormalities.
- Mental retardation.
- Deafness.
- Seventh nerve palsy.
- Coloboma.
- Sporadic, may have chromosome-22 deletion.

Lenz microphthalmia syndrome
- Colobomatous or non-colobomatous microphthalmos.
- Mild mental retardation.
- Prominent ears.
- X-linked recessive.

Goltz syndrome
- Focal dermal hypoplasia.
- X-linked dominant.

Meckel–Gruber syndrome
- Renal abnormalities.
- Occipital encephalocoele.
- Coloboma.
- Autosomal recessive.

Joubert's syndrome
- Coloboma.
- Retinal dystrophy.
- Mental retardation.
- Cerebellar vermis hypoplasia.
- Autosomal recessive.

Warburg's syndrome
- Hydrocephalus.
- Severe brain defects.
- +/− encephalocoele.
- Retinal dysplasia.
- Autosomal recessive.

Coloboma associated with systemic abnormalities of unknown aetiology
Epidermal naevus syndrome
(Fuerstein–Mimms syndrome)
- Mental retardation.
- Non-dermatomal skin pigmentation.

Rubinstein–Taybi syndrome
- Broad thumbs.
- Dysmorphic.
- Mental retardation.

Goldenhar's syndrome
- Lid coloboma.
- Epibulbar dermoid.
- Ear abnormalities.

Miscellaneous
Coloboma with brain defects
- Dandy–Walker cysts.
- Basal encephalocoele.
- Arrhinencephaly.

Teratogens
- Thalidomide.
- Retinoic acid.
- Alcohol.
- Cocaine.

Optic neuropathies

Childhood optic neuritis
Presentation
Sudden unilateral or bilateral visual loss—if unilateral, as strabismus. Ataxia either due to blindness or associated neurological disease.

Visual loss is profound with a central scotoma or diffuse field loss, defective colour vision, an afferent pupil defect and swollen optic discs with few haemorrhages (Fig. 18.20).

Causes
Usually unknown. May be associated with systemic infections such as varicella or it may occur after vaccination.

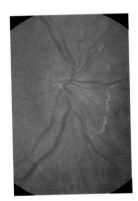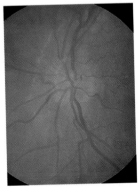

Fig. 18.20 Optic neuritis in a 7-year-old boy. Sudden onset of visual loss to 6/24 acuity right, 1/60 left eye, central scotomas and colour vision loss: bilaterally swollen optic discs. Complete resolution occurred 2 months later.

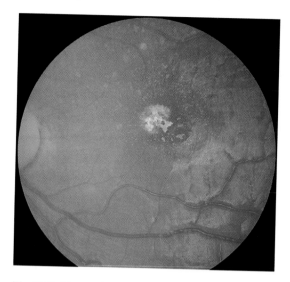

Fig. 18.21 Neuroretinitis. This is a form of optic neuropathy with involvement of the intraocular ganglion cell axons. There is the remains of a macular star—the acuity is 6/9.

Prognosis

The visual prognosis is generally good with full recovery of vision in many cases even if there is a residual optic atrophy. Recovery time is variable, from a few days to several weeks.

Investigations

The VEPs are delayed and have an abnormal amplitude and waveform in the acute stage but may return to normal. CT scanning is usually normal, but MRI may show widespread brain inflammation. This does not necessarily carry a worse prognosis.

Retrobulbar neuritis

This effectively is optic neuritis occurring behind the optic disc and is the same as optic neuritis but without the swollen optic disc.

Neuroretinitis

This may effectively be optic neuritis occurring in

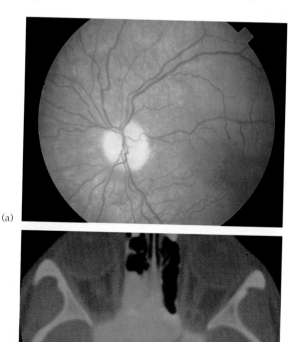

(a)

(c)

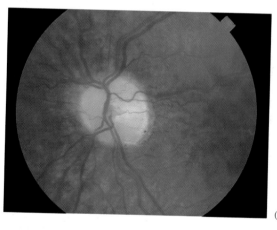

(b)

Fig. 18.22 Fibrous dysplasia. Bilateral optic atrophy. These pictures show the left eye before (a) and after (b) optic nerve decompression. The CT scan (c) shows marked bone thickening and increase in density.

the axons within the eye and is associated with similar symptoms but with a macular star (the prognosis is good) (Fig. 18.21).

Treatment

Systemic steroids in high dose may reduce the length of the attack but it is probably only indicated in bilateral cases.

Optic neuropathy in paranasal sinus disease

Because sphenoid sinusitis or ethmoiditis may give rise to an optic neuropathy, it is important to X-ray the sinuses in most cases of optic neuritis.

Optic neuropathy in leukaemia and systemic neoplasms

This serious complication occurs mostly in acute lymphoblastic leukaemia in relapse. It may also occur with neuroblastoma.

Compressive optic neuropathy

A compressive optic neuropathy may occur with bone disease, i.e. craniometaphyseal dysplasia, fibrous dysplasia (Fig. 18.22) and osteopetrosis. It may occur due to a sphenoid sinus mucocoele or bone infiltration with, for instance, neuroblastoma.

Traumatic optic neuropathy

Blunt trauma may cause a functional optic nerve transection by compression, by the formation of a haematoma or by an associated fracture.

Ischaemic optic neuropathy

This is rare in childhood but occurs with hypertension, especially when the blood pressure is lowered too rapidly, vasculitis and in anomalous discs of anaemic patients.

Toxic optic neuropathies

- Antituberculus drugs.
- Desferrioxamine.
- Cardiac drugs.
- Hydroxyquinolines.
- Antibiotics.
- Antineoplastic agents.

Hereditary optic neuropathies

Dominant optic atrophy (Fig. 18.23)

This is inherited as an autosomal dominant trait with variable expression. New mutations are probably frequent. The onset is insidious, the acuity is 6/9–6/24, rarely worse. Red/green colour vision is normal but blue/yellow may be abnormal. VEPs are normal or show slightly reduced amplitude — the acuity may slowly deteriorate but this is not marked. Field testing shows only very subtle centrocaecal defects. On subjective testing only the peripheral visual field is full. Nystagmus does not occur.

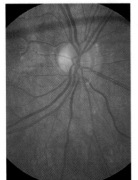
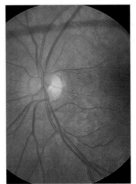
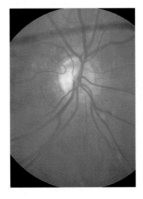
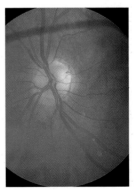

(a)

(b)

Fig. 18.23 (a) Dominant optic atrophy in a 6 year old: he had failed the school test because his acuity was 6/12. He has normal red/green discrimination but defective blue/yellow. (b) The optic discs of the asymptomatic mother of the boy in (a). She had 6/9 acuity in both eyes.

The optic disc is white especially in the temporal segment.

Leber's optic neuropathy

This usually presents in the late teens to 30s with bilateral asynchronous loss of central vision with a time course of a few days or weeks. There is profound acuity loss up to 1/60 or worse; improvement occurs especially with certain mutations. There is a presymptomatic telangiectatic microangiopathy (dilated telangiectatic peripapillary capillaries) (Fig. 18.24). In the acute phase the nerve fibre bundles become swollen. Males are mainly, but not exclusively, affected. It is associated with a number of point mutations of mitochondrial deoxyribonucleic acid (DNA) (11 778, 14 484, 3460). Visual recovery most frequent in patients with the 14 484 and 3460 mutations.

Optic atrophy in juvenile diabetes

The Wolfram–Tyrer syndrome or DIDMOAD (diabetes insipidus, diabetes mellitus, optic atrophy, deafness):
• optic atrophy between 2 and 24 years with severe visual defects (Fig. 18.25);
• juvenile diabetes mellitus of early onset;

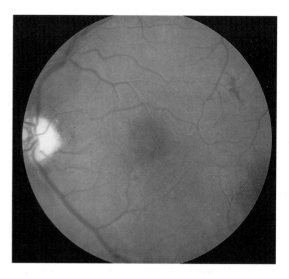

Fig. 18.25 DIDMOAD. Bilateral optic atrophy with profound visual loss.

• diabetes insipidus—usually mild;
• bilateral high-tone deafness;
• pigmentary retinal changes;
• anosmia;
• autosomal recessive.

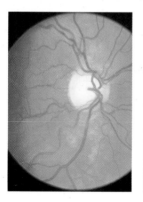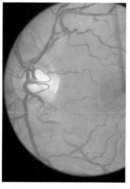

Fig. 18.24 This 14-year-old boy had optic atrophy with a large central scotoma in the right eye which was present for 2 months when he noticed a field defect in the left eye. The left optic disc shows thickened neurones and a peripapillary telangiectatic microangiopathy in the inferotemporal arcades which did not, at the onset, leak fluorescein. His brother and uncle were also affected by Leber's optic neuropathy.

Box 18.3 Swollen optic disc in diabetic children

• Transient papilloedema with visual loss and ensuing optic atrophy with good visual prognosis may occur as a result of optic disc ischaemia.
• Severe hypertension in diabetic retinopathy.
• Raised intracranial pressure due to sinus thrombosis or infections.

Recessive optic atrophy

This is very rare and it is important to exclude retinal disease including the use of ERG to avoid misdiagnosis

Chiasmal disease

Chiasmal disease is characterized by:
1 bitemporal hemianopia;

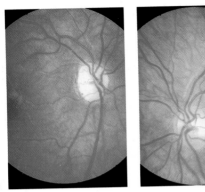
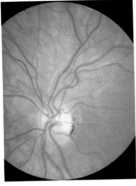

(a)

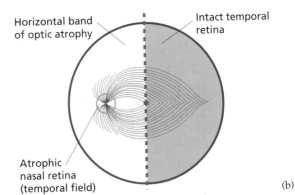

(b)

Fig. 18.26 (a) Craniopharyngioma. The right eye has bare perception of hand movements but the left has an absolute temporal hemianopia, normal colour vision and 6/5 acuity. The left optic disc shows band atrophy—there is all-round loss of the nerve fibres that subserve the defunct temporal visual field but there is preservation of those fibres that subserve the intact nasal field which are inserted into the upper and lower segments of the optic disc. (b) Shows that the margin of the band atrophy is due to the fact that the horizontal band or bow-tie area is the visible area of atrophy where temporal fields for fibres are not inserted into the disc.

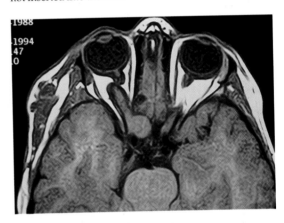

Fig. 18.27 Optic glioma. MRI scan of left optic glioma extending into the chiasm. (Courtesy of Dr Kling Chong and Dr Bob Zimmerman of the Children's Hospital, Philadelphia.)

2 reduced acuity and colour vision in anterior or widespread lesions involving the optic nerves;
3 nystagmus especially see-saw;
4 optic atrophy, characteristically band atrophy (Fig. 18.26);
5 hypothalamic and pituitary disorders;
6 visual complaints due to the bitemporal hemianopia and acuity defects.

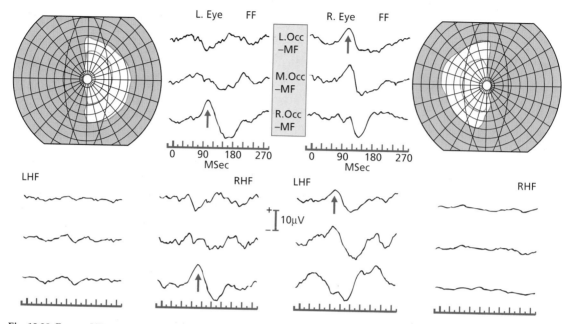

Fig. 18.28 Pattern VEPs of a patient with a bitemporal hemianopia who had been operated for removal of a craniopharyngioma. Note the opposite occipital distribution when comparing full-field stimulation of each eye (crossed asymmetry), and the preserved nasal field responses on half-field stimulation; P100 (arrow) is on the side of scalp ipsilateral to the preserved half-field.

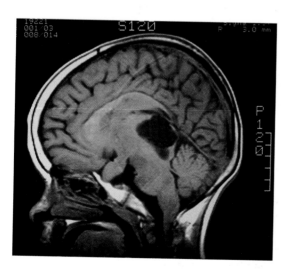

Fig. 18.29 MRI scan of an optic nerve and chiasmal glioma.

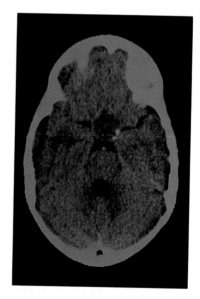

Fig. 18.30 MRI scan of a large cystic craniopharyngioma with calcification in its wall.

Investigation

1 Full clinical investigation especially acuity, fields, colour vision.
2 Neuroimaging.
3 Neurophysiology (Fig. 18.27).

Causes

Developmental defects

The chiasm is hypoplastic in anophthalmia, optic nerve hypoplasia or aplasia. Achiasmia occurs in association with severe developmental defects.

Trauma

Head trauma occasionally produces a sharply defined bitemporal hemianopia or other chiasmal defects.

Tumours

Optic glioma

Optic gliomas are low-grade gliomas that may involve the optic nerve alone, optic nerve and chiasm, chiasm alone or chiasm and hypothalamus. There is a strong association with neurofibromatosis type 1.

Presentation –
• Nystagmus (see-saw).
• Poor vision.
• Growth failure or excessively rapid growth.
• Effects of hydrocephalus resulting from third ventricular involvement.
• Head bobble—a peculiar articulated head movement which occurs usually when the child has hydrocephalus.

Diagnosis and assessment—
1 CT or MRI scanning shows a tube-like thickening of the optic nerve, the chiasm, a suprasellar tumour with contiguous optic nerve expansion and a suprasellar tumour with optic tract involvement. Cystic areas may occur (Figs 18.28 & 18.29).
2 Neurophysiology to assess and document the chiasmal defect. Neurophysiology is particularly useful when one optic nerve is involved in a child because measurements can be made to docu-

ment any damage to the crossing fibres at the chiasm.

Malignant transformation is rare. The tumours are benign and may be hamartomatous.

Treatment—
1 Many exhibit such slow growth that no treatment is necessary.
2 Optic gliomas may be totally resected if vision is very poor, the chiasm is uninvolved or if it has very marked proptosis.
3 These tumours need to be monitored every few months or years depending on the apparent growth rate of the tumour. If vision or hypothalamic function is significantly compromised the patient may be treated with chemotherapy or collimated radiotherapy.
4 Surgery is not indicated except to treat hydrocephalus or to biopsy (which can be done be stereotactic techniques) cases where there is serious doubts about the diagnosis. Occasionally, aspiration of cystic areas may be indicated.

Craniopharyngioma

These present at any age of life and classically present with visual loss or hypothalamic disturbance or hydrocephalus. Diagnosis is by CT or MRI scanning (Fig. 18.30) and treatment is by surgery with or without radiotherapy.

Dysgerminoma

This presents as a classic triad:
1 chiasmal defect;
2 diabetes insipidus;
3 hypothalamic–pituitary disturbances.
    The tumours are often small.
    Other diseases which may affect the chiasm are:
• granulomas;
• Langerhan's cell hystiocytosis;
• tuberculous meningitis;
• sphenoid sinus mucocoele;
• chiasmal neuritis;
• third ventricular distention in hydrocephalus;
• vascular anomalies;
• empty sella syndrome.

19: Posterior Visual Pathways

Brain problems are very important in the context of the child who has vision and other eye problems because:

1 additional defects multiply, not just add onto existing defects;

2 compensation for visual defects is reduced in visually impaired children;

3 education is much more difficult if the child is both visually and mentally handicapped;

4 if seizures are present, medication, the seizures themselves and the associated conditions can compound the problems;

5 affected children also have a wide range of cognitive disorders.

Developmental anomalies

Neuronal migration defects

Lissencephaly (agyria)
• Affected patients may have widespread developmental defects and seizures.
• Neurones fail to migrate giving absence of cortical gyrae (Fig. 19.1).

Pachygyria
Reduced number of gyrae (Fig. 19.2).

Polymicrogyria
Small gyrae with reduced cortical layers (Fig. 19.3). The patients may have focal disorders such as a homonymous hemianopia, or they may be more widespread.

Heterotopias
Neuronal migratory disturbance, usually with periventricular or other aggregations of functionless neuronal material (Fig. 19.4).

Brain cleavage defects
Holoprosencephaly
In this condition there is one degree or another of single cerebral ventricle usually with other abnormal brain structures. There may be associated facial defects, midline clefts or nose defects. Microcephaly is frequent and agenesis of the corpus callosum often occurs (Fig. 19.4). Optic nerve hypoplasia may be associated with this condition (see Chapter 18).

Schizencephaly
These are variable clefts in the brain substance with free communication or a grey matter track between ventricles and the subarachnoid space.

Porencephaly
Insults to the brain in later fetal life result in defects affecting variable proportions of the brain. The occipital lobe is often affected. Porencephalic cysts often correspond to a territory perfused by a cerebral vessel (Fig. 19.5).

Colpocephaly
The cause is unclear but there are unilateral or bilateral dilatations of the occipital horns of the ventricles. Optic disc associations may be associated and vision can be severely compromised by the cortical defect.

Congenital vascular anomalies
For example, Sturge–Weber syndrome (see Chapter 24).

Acquired brain disorders affecting vision

Hypoxic/ischaemic encephalopathy
• Perinatal asphyxia.
• Cardiorespiratory arrests.

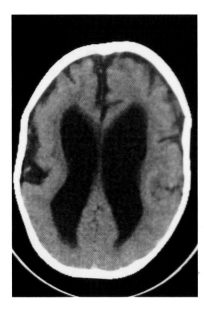

Fig. 19.1 Agyria, a severe form of lissencephaly. On this computerized tomography scan it can be seen that the surface of the brain posteriorly is smooth. The rest of the brain is atrophic shown by large sulci and ventricles.

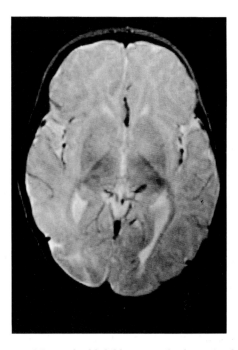

Fig. 19.3 A 9-month-old child was noted to have visual inattention to the left at the age of 6 weeks by her mother. At 9 months of age the hemianopia was more difficult to detect clinically, but visual evoked potentials recorded from the two hemispheres were grossly symmetrical. The magnetic resonance imaging scan shows hypoplasia of the right occipital lobe. The child was the product of a full-term uncomplicated pregnancy and delivery. She is developmentally normal otherwise. The smaller size of the right occipital pole can be seen.

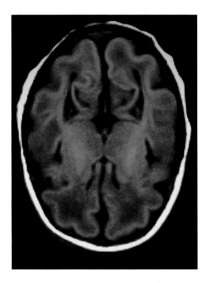

Fig. 19.2 Pachygyria. This disorder is similar to lissencephaly and shows the true form and smoothness of the gyri.

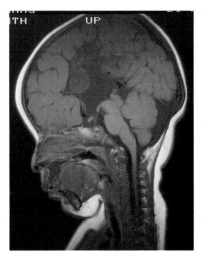

Fig. 19.4 Aicardi's syndrome showing agenesis of the corpus collusum and neuronal heterotopia.

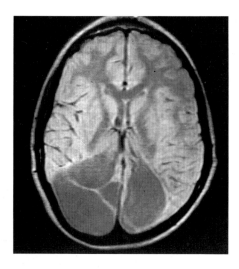

Fig. 19.5 Bilateral porencephalic cysts.

- Near-miss cot death.
- Near drowning.
- Intraoperative asphyxia.

Watershed infarcts

These are infarcts between vascular zones, i.e. between the posterior cerebral artery and the middle cerebral artery in the occipital cortex, or in the parasagittal zones in premature infants. A watershed zone is in the periventricular region.

Hypoxic ischaemic damage results in loss of cerebral substance with atrophy, enlarged sulci and ventricles.

Generalized brain atrophy

Periventricular leucomalacia in premature babies

Periventricular haemorrhage occurs in many sick, small, premature infants. It results from ischaemic damage to the subependymal layer with a resulting haemorrhage, which may damage the brain substance. This may result in severe damage to the posterior visual pathway (Fig. 19.6) and give rise to a wide variety of cerebral and other defects, including tonic downward gaze, esotropia and visual defects.

Trauma

Trauma may affect the visual cortex directly or by contracoup. It is frequently secondary to non-accidental injury (see Chapter 25). The severity of the brain injury in non-accidental injury may be reflected by the extent of any retinal haemorrhages. Initially, there is haemorrhage and oedema resulting in neuronal damage, atrophy and gliosis (Fig. 19.7).

Meningitis

Haemophilus influenzae, meningococcal and pneumococcal meningitis frequently cause deafness and blindness. *Haemophilus* may have a predilection for the occipital cortex. Tuberculous meningitis may occasionally damage the visual cortex.

Metabolic disease

Leigh's disease, X-linked adrenoleucodystrophy and many other neurometabolic diseases (see Chapter 20) may cause cerebral visual defects.

Hydrocephalus

Aetiology

1 *Developmental defects*:
   (a) aqueduct stenosis;
   (b) Arnold–Chiari malformations;
   (c) spina bifida, meningomyelocoele;
   (d) other developmental abnormalities, i.e. arachnoid cysts.

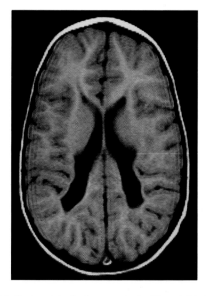

Fig. 19.6 Periventricular leucomalacia. T1-weighted sequence in a 3-year-old boy who was substantially premature and had periventricular haemorrhages in the newborn period.

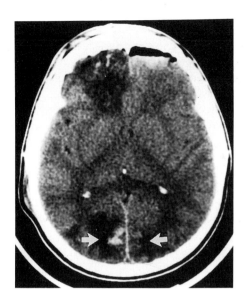

Fig. 19.7 Axial computerized tomography scan of a youth who fell off a cliff and landed on his face. There is a contracoup contusion injury in both occipital lobes with oedema and haemorrhage involving the visual cortex (arrows). The patient had no light perception for 1 week, but by 2 weeks his vision had returned to normal. There is also a frontal lesion.

2 *Acquired lesions*:
  (a) meningitis;
  (b) intracranial haemorrhage — especially in premature infants;
  (c) infections
      (i) congenital toxoplasmosis
      (ii) meningitis;
  (d) tumours.
3 *Fourth ventricle and aqueduct abnormalities —* medulloblastoma, astrocytoma and ependymoma.
4 *Third ventricle*:
  (a) optic chiasm glioma;
  (b) craniopharyngioma;
  (c) arachnoid cyst.

Presenting symptoms and signs
1 *Infancy*:
  (a) enlarging head;
  (b) tense fontanelle;
  (c) dilated scalp veins;
  (d) upgaze palsy with lid retraction (setting-sun sign) (Fig. 19.8);

  (e) papilloedema—rare;
  (f) irritability;
  (g) if marked, cerebral loss gives rise to transillumination (Fig. 19.9).
2 *Childhood onset*:
  (a) headaches;
  (b) early morning vomiting which relieves headaches;
  (c) bilateral papilloedema;

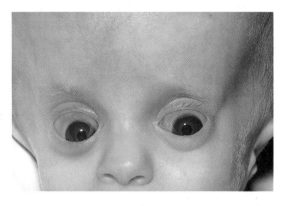

Fig. 19.8 Setting-sun sign. This consists of a downward deviation of the eyes, an upgaze palsy and lid retraction.

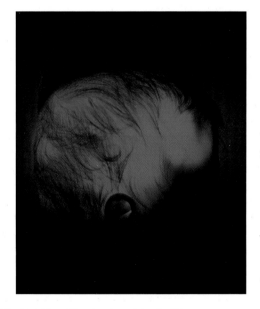

Fig. 19.9 Transillumination of the skull in severe hydrocephalus.

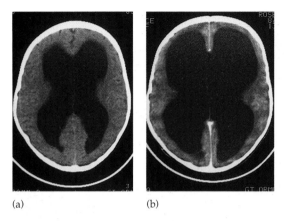

(a)   (b)

Fig. 19.10 Hydrocephalus. (a) The ventricles are huge with a thin cortical mantle. (b) The same child after ventriculoatrial shunting.

(d) bilateral sixth nerve palsy or concomitant esotropia;

(e) vertical gaze impairment.

Diagnosis and investigation
1 *Imaging*.
  (a) Ultrasound — this can be done in children before the fontanelle has closed and gives a reasonable view of the ventricular size and much of the brain substance.
  (b) Computerized tomography (CT) and magnetic resonance imaging (MRI) scanning (Fig. 19.10) — these may detail the size of the ventricle, the presence of cerebral atrophy and any associated masses or developmental defects. Repeat scanning may be required.
  (c) Intracranial pressure measurement:
    (i) lumbar puncture (after CT scanning. Should not be carried out in the presence of large ventricles);
    (ii) transcranial monitoring — good for patients with dubiously raised intracranial pressure, i.e. craniosynostoses, long-standing hydrocephalus with large head, etc., and where there may be diurnal variations in intracranial pressure.

Treatment of hydrocephalus
1 Treatment of the cause.
2 Shunting.

Ocular complications of hydrocephalus
1 *Optic atrophy*:
  (a) secondary to papilloedema;
  (b) secondary to third ventricular compression of the chiasm and optic nerve;
  (c) associated with causative tumours, i.e. optic glioma, periventricular leucomalacia;
  (d) in prenatal hydrocephalus, trans-synaptic optic nerve degeneration may occur.
2 *Eye movement defects*.
  (a) Concomitant strabismus:
    (i) 'A' pattern esotropia most frequent with the deviation being greater for distance than for near;
    (ii) bilateral superior oblique overaction frequent (Fig. 19.11).
  (b) Strabismus associated with visual defect — this is often divergent, exotropia.
  (c) Bilateral sixth nerve palsies — often partial.
  (d) Third nerve palsies.
  (e) Bilateral fourth nerve palsies — with hydrocephalus and posterior fossa pathology.
  (f) Gaze palsies:
    (i) these occur especially in young infants (setting-sun sign);
    (ii) older children with posterior fossa problems may have vertical or occasionally horizontal gaze palsies.
  (g) Nystagmus — usually related to visual loss or associated chiasmal disease.

Ophthalmological follow-up
Where possible, all children who have had hydrocephalus that has not clearly and definitely undergone spontaneous resolution or has resolved following treatment (i.e. meningitis) should, where possible, have a follow-up not only by the neurosurgeon but also by an ophthalmologist who needs to take an account of visual acuity, colour vision and visual fields together with examination of the optic discs. Where available, neurophysiological studies may be helpful. Some children with refractory hydrocephalus pose very difficult problems in ophthalmological follow-up. Because of the difficulty in eliciting signs and very poor vision, detection of changes from one visit to another may be very difficult.

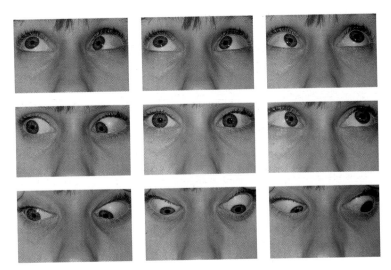

Fig. 19.11 'A' pattern esotropia in a child with hydrocephalus. Note the overaction of the superior oblique muscles.

Box 19.1 Headaches in children

1 Stress headaches.
2 Hypertension.
3 Raised intracranial pressure.
4 Low intracranial pressure.
5 Eye and ocular motor disease.
6 Periocular causes—bone and sinus disease.
7 Meningism and meningitis.
8 Post-traumatic.
9 Migraine.
10 Hypoglycaemia.
11 Fever.
12 Nerve entrapment, i.e. bone dysplasias or tumours.
13 Temporomandibular arthritis in children with bone or craniofacial disease.

Assessment of cerebral defects

Clinical

Ophthalmological evaluation

Visual field studies, estimation of acuity, colour vision and evaluation of eye movements and strabismus are helpful in all cases, together with examination of the fundi, especially for optic atrophy and papilloedema. Small children need simpler methods (see Chapter 4).

Neurological evaluation

This will take into account associated neurological defects such as seizures, intellectual impairment, spasticity and movement defects, monitoring of head size, etc.

Psychological evaluation

Psychological evaluation may be very helpful for intellectual and educational assessment, and for the monitoring of any progressive intellectual impairment such as may occur in chronic mildly raised intracranial pressure (craniosynostoses).

Scanning

MRI scanning is the most helpful in looking at grey and white matter, myelin development, the posterior fossa and the chiasmal region to help delineate structural defects and observe changes with time.

CT scanning is also helpful especially when bone abnormalities are present, or when it is most important to outline brain calcification.

Neurophysiology

Electroencephalography (EEG)

This may be helpful, especially to detect seizure activity, other focal abnormalities and specific patterns, i.e. hypsarrhythmia, etc.

Visual neurophysiology

Visual evoked potentials (VEPs) may help to determine prognosis. If even flash VEPs are not present, good recovery is less likely, whilst if small check-pattern responses are present then at least primary visual cortical activation is likely and the more favourable visual recovery is possible.

VEPs may be normal despite severe visual defect if other brain areas are damaged.

Electroretinograms (ERGs) may be helpful to exclude associated retinal disease.

Vision in brain-damaged infants and children

Ophthalmological vision and other measurements

1 *Acuity*. Visual acuity for near and distance is often difficult to measure in brain-damaged children because of associated defects. Acuity may be variably abnormal depending on the severity of the brain defect and any associated defect.

2 *Colour vision* is usually unaffected unless there is an associated colour agnosia (see below).

3 *Visual fields*. Unilateral tract optic radiation and occipital cortex defects give rise to homonymous hemianopias. These may be bilateral, the extent of the defect varying with the extent of the disease. Testing may be very difficult in these children, compounded by attentional defects, behaviour and intellectual problems.

4 The eyes are basically normal and the pupil reactions are normal in brain problems unless there are associated anterior visual system disorders.

5 *Nystagmus and eye movement disorders* are infrequent in brain disorders unless basal ganglia or the brainstem is also involved.

Attentional defects

Half-field inattention

Children with this condition will tend to ignore objects on one side. Visual field testing is very difficult but needs to take into account reflexive eye movements into the half-field that the patient has inattention to. They are usually unaware of the condition.

Generalized inattention

Generalized inattention shows itself as a child's inability to recognise familiar objects, i.e. his or her parents, siblings, friends, etc. A clinical clue may be given by the child apparently seeing better when he

or she also hears or touches the object which he or she otherwise ignores. A classic situation is the child running along in an open and uncrowded area and not recognizing his or her parent who is in that area until they say something.

Visual agnosias

Prosopagnosia

This right posterior hemisphere associated defect results in patients being unable to recognize faces despite good vision.

Object agnosia

Despite good vision and the ability to distinguish detail and understand dimensions the patient is unable to perceive the meaning of various objects, sometimes even in spite of an ability to draw them. This must be distinguished from an inability to name the object.

Topographic agnosia

Despite good vision the patient has difficulty in finding their way around, sometimes even in familiar territory. They may need to use other visual cues to navigate successfully.

Colour agnosia

Despite good acuity and an ability to detect subtle coloured objects such as Ishihara plates, the patient has poor subjective colour vision.

Simultagnosia

Despite good vision the patient is unable to take in more than one object in a visual field at a time. Patients may not be able to pay attention to objects lying either side of the fixation point. It is due to bilateral occipital lobe lesions.

Balint's syndrome is due to bilateral parieto-occipital lobe lesions:
1 simultagnosia;
2 supranuclear paralysis of gaze;
3 motor problems, in particular past-pointing, particularly with the right hand.

Anosognosia

An inability to recognise the presence of an agnosia or other disorder.

Palinopsia

- Evolving right parietal lesions.
- Associated field defect.
- 'Visual perseveration in time' — patients perceive an object which they have already seen and which they return to in a stereotype fashion on several occasions over a period of time.

Blindsight and extrageniculostriate vision

It is proposed that neonates and young infants have visual responses mediated by a non-striate visual system—the extrageniculate striate system which, it is proposed, is a 'primitive visual system'. In several situations there is evidence of residual extragenicular striate function. Blindsight is a preservation of visual function in a defective visual field, usually a homonymous hemianopia associated with occipital disease. Patients may show reflex, eye movements and an ability to perceive movement and some static stimuli in the apparently blind half-field. It is suggested that a form of blindsight may be responsible for children with severe cerebral blindness, having relatively good navigational skills, but it is very difficult to exclude residual striate vision as the mechanism for this.

20: Neurometabolic Disease

Neurometabolic diseases or the neurolipidoses are a group of inherited errors of metabolism affecting the nervous system, amongst which eye signs are very prominent. Since the ophthalmologist looks directly not only at vascular elements, but also at neurones, the highly metabolic pigment epithelium and the choroid it is perhaps not surprising that eye signs are protean.

Gangliosidoses

GM1 gangliosidoses
Infantile GM1 type I
- β-galactosidase deficiency.
- Visceral involvement: liver, spleen and kidney enlargement.
- Coarse features, Hurler-like.
- Cherry red spots.
- Cerebral degeneration, occasional seizures.
- Regression and death by 2 years.
- Corneal clouding.
- Autosomal recessive.

Late infantile GM1 type II
- Mental and motor regression.
- Normal facial features.
- Seizures.
- Kyphoscoliosis.
- Autosomal recessive.

Clinical Tay–Sachs disease, Tay–Sachs (GM2 type I), Sandhoffs (GM2 type II)
- Tay–Sachs: hexosaminidase A deficient.
- Sandhoffs: hexosaminidase A and B deficient.
- Regression in first year of life.
- Exaggerated startle response to sound and light.
- Head enlargement.
- Cherry red spot leading to optic atrophy.

- Death by 4 years of age.
- Autosomal recessive.

Batten's disease (neuronal ceroid lipofuscinosis)

Four main forms of Batten's disease occur. All have retinal degeneration, regression and seizures; the juvenile form is most frequently seen by ophthalmologists.

Juvenile Batten's disease
Also known as Batten–Mayou disease, Vogt–Spielmeyer disease, Spielmeyer–Sjögren disease and juvenile neuronal ceroid lipofuscinosis.
- Visual loss is the first symptom with an onset between 4 and 10 years.
- Bull's eye maculopathy (Fig. 20.1).
- Eccentric viewing, patients tend to hold eyes in upgaze, using lower field, i.e. 'overlooking'.
- Later, the whole retina is affected.
- Electroretinograph (ERG) abnormal, B wave attenuated first.
- Blindness within 3 years.
- Mental deterioration and behavioural problems around the time of the visual deterioration.
- Gradual loss of skills and regression with death by the age of up to 25 years.
- Seizures between 7 and 16 years of age.
- The seizures are not usually difficult to control.
- Autosomal recessive.

Diagnosis
1 Vaculated lymphocytes in peripheral blood smears (Fig. 20.2).
2 Fingerprint inclusions on electron microscopy studies of rectal biopsies, skin, conjunctiva or lymphocyte.

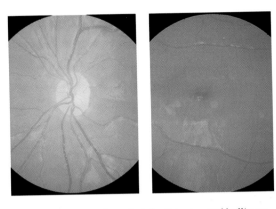

Fig. 20.1 Optic atrophy, arteriolar thinning and bull's eye maculopathy in juvenile Batten's disease.

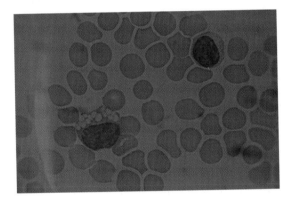

Fig. 20.2 Juvenile Batten's disease—lymphocyte inclusions.

Niemann–Pick disease

Group 1

Infantile, juvenile and adult forms occur. The infantile form is most common. This group is sphingomyelinase deficient.

Type A: neurovisceral, infantile
- Onset first 6 months of life.
- Hepatosplenomegaly.
- Regression.
- Cherry red spots (Fig. 20.3).
- Optic atrophy later.
- Autosomal recessive.

Type B: visceral
- Later onset more frequent.

- Occasional mild cherry red spots.
- Massive visceromegaly.
- Pulmonary and bone marrow infiltration.

Group 2

This group is sphyngomyelinase normal.

Type C: variable onset
1 Infancy with liver dysfunction, jaundice and psychomotor deterioration, early death.
2 Four to six years intellectual deterioration, vertical supranuclear palsy, ataxia.
3 Adolescent form.

The most common abnormality seen by ophthalmologists in this group is in those with an onset of about 6 years where they develop a vertical supranuclear palsy (Fig. 20.4), in particular with loss of vertical saccades, especially downwards, and the preservation of doll's eye movements. A cherry red spot has been observed. The diagnosis is made by the finding of foamy macrophages in bone marrow and membrane-bound polymorphous concentrically multilamellated cytoplastic bodies in neurones. It is autosomal recessive.

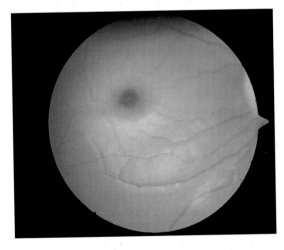

Fig. 20.3 Cherry red spots in an Asian patient with Neimann–Pick type A: the spot is red because of dark background pigmentation. The spot itself is normal, it is the opalescence surrounding the retina due to ganglion cell involvement that causes the spot to appear relatively red.

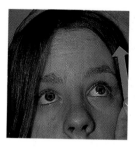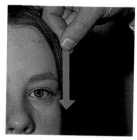

Fig. 20.4 Downgaze palsy in a child with Neimann–Pick type C. The arrow denotes the direction that the child is being told to look. Horizontal and upgaze were normal.

Type D
- Very rare.
- Similar to type C.
- Found in Nova Scotia.

Gaucher's disease

- Glucocerebrosidase deficient.
- 'Gaucher' cells in many tissues.
- Autosomal recessive.

Type I
- Chronic hepatosplenomegaly.
- Pingueculae.
- Rarely, central nervous system degeneration.
- Rarely, macularhalo.
- Later onset.

Type II
- Infantile onset.
- Delayed development, regression, death by 2 years.
- Seizures.
- Cherry red spots.

Type III
- Onset birth to 14 years.
- Intellectual deterioration, seizures.
- Vertical supranuclear palsy.
- Strabismus.

Neuraminidase deficiency

Sialidosis type I: cherry red spot–myoclonus syndrome
- Cherry red spots, insidious visual loss.
- Progressive myoclonus.

Sialidosis type II
- Hurler's phenotype.
- Regression.
- Corneal clouding, cherry red spot.

Box 20.1   Eye movement disorders in neurometabolic disease

- Vertical gaze palsy ('apraxia'):
  (a) Niemann–Pick type C;
  (b) Gaucher's disease.
- Nystagmus:
  (a) sialidosis type I;
  (b) Canavan's disease;
  (c) Pelizaeus–Merzbacher disease;
  (d) all conditions that cause blindness.
- Chaotic eye movements:
  (a) organic acidaemias;
  (b) urea cycle disorders;
  (c) Leigh's disease.
- Strabismus: most cases with visual defect.

The mucopolysaccharidoses

Although the paediatric ophthalmologist was rarely involved with these conditions (Table 20.1), their survival as a result of bone marrow transplantation makes ophthalmological involvement more frequent.

They have features in common, but which are not present in all cases.

Table 20.1 The mucopolysaccharidoses.

MPS IH	Hurler	AR
MPS IS	Scheie	AR
MPS II	Hunter	X-LR
MPS III	Sanfilippo	AR
MPS IVA	Morquio	AR
MPS VI	Maroteaux–Lamy	AR
MPS VII	Sly	AR

Corneal clouding

The corneas are thickened and diffusely infiltrated with glycosaminoglycans in the cells, in the stroma and in the extracellular space. The cornea is homogeneously cloudy (Fig. 20.5). Clouding can clear with bone marrow transplantation at least partially and, if severe, can be treated by corneal transplantation but the cornea itself is often not the main cause of any vision defect. It is unusual in Hunter's and mild in Sanfilippo's.

Retinal degeneration

This is seen in all forms, except Morquio's disease, and is usually only detectable by ERG as the retina cannot usually be seen because of the corneal clouding. The onset of symptoms is insidious, often starting with difficulty with night vision.

Optic neuropathy

An optic neuropathy occurs mainly due to direct infiltration with glycosaminoglycans, but there may also be some cases in whom there is bilateral papilloedema with or without evidence of raised intracranial pressure. This may be due to a very thickened sclera causing compression at the optic nerve head. Optic neuropathy is rare in Sanfilippo's and Morquio's. Optic atrophy can also be caused by glaucoma.

Glaucoma

Glaucoma is quite frequent and needs to be

screened for and is due to glycosaminoglycans in the drainage channels. The cloudy corneas may make diagnosis and management difficult.

The ophthalmologist's role in the management of patients with mucopolysaccharidoses

1 Make sure that their vision cannot be improved by glasses or low-vision appliances.
2 Corneal transplantation may be helpful after the exclusion of retinal degeneration, glaucoma or optic neuropathy.
3 Check for glaucoma or the presence of optic atrophy.
4 Detect papilloedema if present, and help manage the raised intracranial pressure either by medications, shunting or optic nerve fenestration.
5 Monitor changes in the cornea, retina, etc., after bone marrow transplantation.
6 Neurophysiological studies may help to define retinal and optic nerve problems, and monitor progression.

Mucolipidoses

These are rare conditions with some features of mucopolysaccharidoses and some of neurolipidoses. From the point of view of the paediatric ophthalmologist only one is important: mucolipidosis IV.

Mucolipidosis IV
• Corneal clouding or corneal verticillata from 18 months.
• The corneal clouding is mainly epithelial.
• Developmental regression with hypotonia and death within a few years.
• Mild forms may occur.
• Retinal degeneration, cataracts.
• Autosomal recessive.

Mannosidosis

• Mild corneal opacity.
• Spoke-like cataract in posterior cortex.
• Coarse facies, bony changes, regression.
• Autosomal recessive.

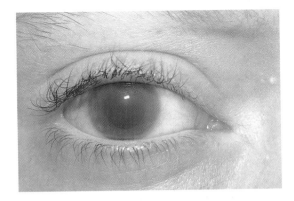

Fig. 20.5 Opaque cornea in a patient with Scheie's MPS IS. The acuity was 6/12.

Fucosidosis

- Mental and motor regression, growth retardation.
- Coarse facies.
- Bone dysplasia.
- Autosomal recessive.
- Conjunctival and retinal vascular tortuosity.
- Bull's eye maculopathy.
- Corneal opacities.

Fabry's disease

- Truncal telangiectases.
- Marked peripheral neuropathy.
- Renal disease.
- Conjunctiva vessel tortuosity.
- Lid oedema.
- Cornea verticillata (Fig. 20.6).
- Lens opacities.
- Nystagmus.
- Optic atrophy.
- X-linked recessive.

Leucodystrophies

Metachromatic leucodystrophy

- Progressive motor and behavioural problems.
- Peripheral neuropathy.
- Primary optic atrophy in one out of three cases.
- Cherry red spot giving rise to optic atrophy.

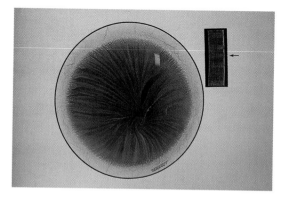

Fig. 20.6 Fabry's disease. A painting of cornea verticillata. Usually the whorled lines are very faint and cannot be seen without slit lamp microscopy.

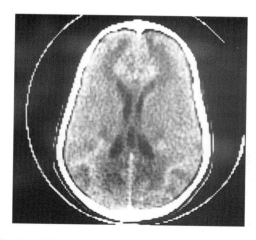

Fig. 20.7 Adrenoleucodystrophy. Periventricular lucency and enhancement on CT scanning.

- Autosomal recessive.
- Diagnosis:
  (a) by finding urinary intracellular metachromatic substances;
  (b) aryl sulphatase deficiency.

Krabbe's disease
- Galactocerebrosidase deficiency.
- Regression in infancy.
- Irritability, failure to thrive.
- Exaggerated startle response.
- Peripheral neuropathy.
- Optic atrophy.
- Cortical blindness.

Adrenoleucodystrophy
- Cortical blindness associated with low-density zones in periventricular white matter posteriorly (Fig. 20.7) on computerized tomography (CT) or magnetic resonance imaging scanning.
- Addison's disease with hyperpigmentation.
- Optic atrophy.
- X-linked recessive.
- Regression and death in a few years.

Organic acidaemias
For example, maple syrup urine disease, propionic acidaemia, glutaric aciduria, etc.
- Metabolic acidosis.

- Rapid deterioration.
- Ketosis.
- Failure to thrive.
- Seizures.
- Gaze paresis.
- Nystagmus.
- Ptosis.

Menke's disease

- X-linked recessive.
- Slow maturation from birth.
- Abnormal hair (feels like wire wool).
- Sparse eyebrows.
- Well-preserved eyelashes.
- Retinal dystrophy with abnormal ERG.
- Tortuous retinal vessels.
- Optic nerve demyelination.

Phenylketonuria

- High refractive errors.

- Cataract.
- Gradual mental retardation.
- Pale rough skin.
- Fair hair and blue eyes.
- Autosomal recessive.

Box 20.2 Cherry red spot

- GM2 types I, II and III.
- GM1 type I.
- Neimann–Pick:
  (a) group 1, types A and B;
  (b) group 2, type C (occasionally Gaucher's disease type II, rarely type I).
- Metachromatic leucodystrophy.
- Farber's disease.
- Mucolipodoses type III.
- Sialidosis types 1 and II.

21: Dyslexia (Specific Learning Disorders)

Academic failure may come about for a number of reasons, few of which have any medical cause. However, certain neurological conditions may have a great impact on academic performance, particularly those associated with mild mental retardation or attention deficit disorders. The term dyslexia has been reserved for the condition in which a specific reading disability exists in a patient with no other evidence of neurological problems, normal intelligence and good general health. Many of these patients are referred to ophthalmologists because of the mistaken notion that a specific ocular, ocular motor or visual 'processing' disorder exists to account for this poor academic performance.

However, careful longitudinal controlled studies have failed to document any specific ophthalmic disorder that occurs with a greater frequency in this affected group compared with age-matched controls. All the following have been examined and have not been found to be specifically associated with dyslexia:

1 strabismus, especially small esotropias or convergence insufficiency;
2 relationship of ocular dominance to handedness;
3 pursuit eye movements;
4 saccadic eye movements;
5 vergence amplitudes;
6 vestibular ocular function;
7 optokinetic nystagmus;
8 dysfunction of the magnocellular ganglion cells.

This is not to say that there may not be a neuropathological correlate for some cases of dyslexia. Indeed, computerized tomography, magnetic resonance imaging and autopsy studies have suggested that in the dyslexic patient a reversal of the normal pattern of cerebral asymmetry occurs such that the right temporoparietal occipital area is larger than the left. Other post-mortem studies have documented neuronal migration anomalies in the left cortex, particularly around the Sylvian fissure and left planum temporale. Foci of ectopic neurones in the subcortical white matter and bilateral abnormalities of the thalamus have also been reported. None of these findings would be expected to lead to a specific disorder of ocular motor dysfunction or processing within the anterior visual pathways. A number of quasi-medical therapies have been advocated for the treatment of the dyslexic patient including:

1 eye movement exercises;
2 antivestibular medications;
3 tinted spectacle lenses;
4 general motor development exercises.

In scientific-controlled studies none of these has been proven to be specifically efficacious in the treatment of the learning disabled patient. That is not, of course, to imply that any abnormality of the visual system in the learning disabled patient should not be corrected, but rather that no direct association with ocular abnormalities and learning disabilities has been documented.

The role of the ophthalmologist, therefore, is usually to examine the patient's visual and ocular motor system and treat any abnormalities, reassure the parents and be a source of information about learning disabilities.

Ultimately, his or her most important role is to reinforce the role of good teaching, and be an advocate for the child and parents who are often extraordinarily distraught because of the problem.

22: Pupil Anomalies and Reactions

Development (Fig. 22.1)

The pupillary light response is absent in infants of 29 gestational weeks or less, but is usually present by 31 or 32 weeks. At birth the pupil is usually small. This is apparently due to reduced sympathetic tone. In very premature babies the pupil may not have fully formed until after 32 weeks' gestation; mydriasis should not be taken as necessarily indicating a central nervous system lesion, nor does an unresponsive pupil necessarily indicate an afferent defect.

Congenital and structural anomalies

Congenital, structural and developmental anomalies of the pupil include the following (see Chapters 13 and 18):

- aniridia;
- micropupil (congenital idiopathic microcoria);
- polycoria and corectopia;
- coloboma;
- persistent pupillary membrane;
- congenital mydriasis and miosis;
- irregular pupils.

Afferent pupillary defect

Amaurotic pupil

A totally blind eye has no pupillary light response. If the blindness is unilateral, the affected eye has no pupil reaction when a light is shone on it, but when the light is shifted into the unaffected eye both pupils rapidly constrict. If both eyes are blind from anterior visual pathway or retinal disease, both pupils are usually dilated if the condition is recent, although they may be nearly normal in size in long-standing blindness. The pupils may remain reactive to an imagined near stimulus.

Relative afferent pupil defect (Marcus Gunn)

The relative afferent pupillary defect is essentially a test of optic nerve function, although it may be abnormal in patients with extensive retinal disease. It never occurs with corneal disease, cataract, moderate-sized vitreous haemorrhage or macular disease. It may occur in some patients with amblyopia.

It is tested for in a dimly lit room. The observer uses a bright light which is shone on each eye individually. The child must maintain fixation in the distance during testing. The light is first shone on the suspected better (normal) eye for a few seconds and then rapidly moved to the suspected worse eye. If the second eye has worse conduction within the pupillomotor fibres both pupils will dilate despite the light stimulus. The relative afferent pupillary defect is a sensitive test, even in children, and it is not uncommon to find a positive response even in the presence of normal acuity and colour vision, particularly in compressive disorders.

A complete optic tract lesion may be associated with a mild contralateral relative afferent pupillary defect, although this is rarely clinically detectable. No relative afferent pupillary defect is associated with chiasmal disease.

Light–near dissociation

When the pupillary response is better to a near rather than a light stimulus, light–near dissociation is said to occur. A bright light is necessary in order to be certain that this is present. This appears to come about as a result of damage to the pupillomotor fibres in the dorsal midbrain after they have branched from the optic tract but before they have become associated with the fibres of the near response in the Edinger–Westphal nucleus.

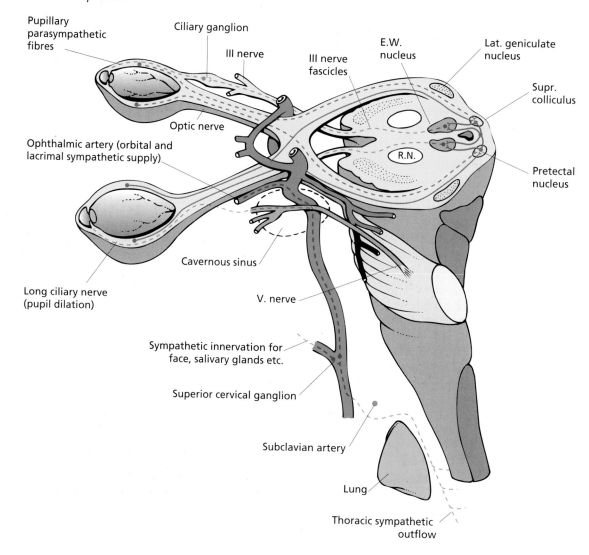

Pupillary
parasympathetic
fibres

Ciliary ganglion

III nerve

III nerve
fascicles

E.W.
nucleus

Lat. geniculate
nucleus

Supr.
colliculus

Optic nerve

Ophthalmic artery (orbital and
lacrimal sympathetic supply)

R.N.

Pretectal
nucleus

Cavernous sinus

Long ciliary nerve
(pupil dilation)

V. nerve

Sympathetic innervation for
face, salivary glands etc.

Superior cervical ganglion

Subclavian artery

Lung

Thoracic sympathetic
outflow

Fig. 22.1 Schematic representation of the efferent and afferent pathways involved in pupillary reactions. Red, blood vessels and parasympathetic system; blue, afferent visual pathways; green, sympathetic pathways. E.W., Edinger–Westphal.

Argyll Robertson pupils

This pupillary condition is characterized by small irregular pupils that constrict more fully and briskly to a near stimulus than to light. They may also dilate less well than normal pupils. The iris is often seen to be atrophic on slit lamp examination. This abnor-

mality is usually seen in adults with tertiary syphilis. It may be seen in young patients with congenital syphilis. The pseudo-Argyll Robertson pupil that has been reported in diabetes is not small and has rarely been reported before the third decade.

Sylvian aqueduct syndrome

Compression of the dorsal midbrain by expanding tumours (pinealomas, ependymomas, trilateral retinoblastomas, granulomas) may produce bilateral light–near dissociation. However, the resting size of the pupil is usually larger than normal.

Other accompanying signs may include vertical gaze palsy, lid retraction, accommodative defects, convergence–retraction nystagmus and strabismus (convergence paralysis).

Segmental or sinus pupil reactions

In some conditions pupillary reactions appear to be segmental or sinuous with one part of the iris sphincter reacting better than another. This may occur in the following.

Adie's syndrome (tonic pupil syndrome)

This condition may occur in children but is more frequently seen in young adults, especially women. It is usually unilateral but is occasionally bilateral. The acutely affected pupil is usually a little larger than its uninvolved fellow, but if viewed in the darkness may be smaller as the normal pupil is free to dilate widely. The involved pupil has segmental paralysis of the iris sphincter with a sluggish and sinuous pupillary response to light thus occurring. There is also a defect in accommodation which is often marked in the acute phase but gradually improves over 1 or 2 years. If the affected child is hyperopic the possibility of anisometropia amblyopia must be recalled.

Other features associated with the tonic pupil include:

- reduced corneal sensation in the involved eye;
- reduced reflexes in the extremities.

Denervation hypersensitivity may be demonstrated in this syndrome by instilling pilocarpine 0.1% or methacholine 2.5% and observing a pupillary response to these weak solutions. The proposed site for this lesion is the ciliary ganglion and a relationship to neurotrophic viruses has been suggested. In children, a particular relationship with chickenpox has been noted (Fig. 22.2).

Other causes of tonic pupil

Other causes of ciliary ganglion damage may give rise to a syndrome similar to Adie's. This has been reported in:

- orbital tumours;
- syphilis;
- diabetes;
- Guillain–Barré syndrome;

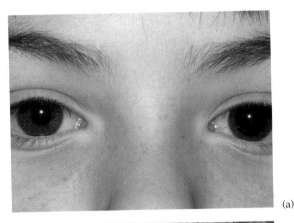

(a)

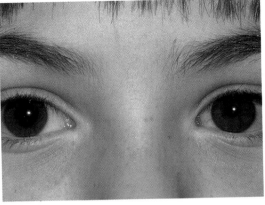

(b)

Fig. 22.2 (a) Left Adie's pupil before bilateral instillation of 0.1% pilocarpine. (b) Left Adie's pupil 20 minutes after instillation of 0.1% pilocarpine. The right pupil is unchanged, the left constricts due to denervation hypersensitivity.

- Miller–Fisher syndrome;
- pandysautonomia;
- hereditary sensory neuropathy;
- Charcot–Marie–Tooth disease;
- trilene poisoning;
- paraneoplastic disease with autonomic neuropathy and chronic relapsing polyneuropathy.

Third nerve palsy (Fig. 22.3)

Complete paresis of the third nerve produces an unresponsive pupil, but in a partial or recovering third nerve palsy the involved pupillary reactions may be sluggish and react unevenly, resulting in a

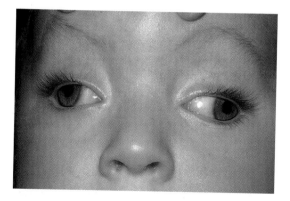

Fig. 22.3 Bilateral congenital third nerve palsy with fixed and unreactive pupils; the pupils made very slow bilateral size changes.

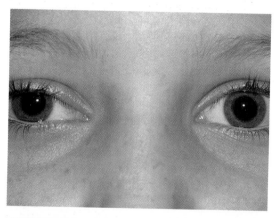

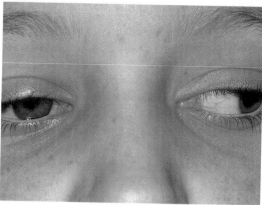

Fig. 22.4 Aberrant regeneration following partial recovery from right traumatic third nerve palsy. The right pupil constricts on attempted abduction.

sinuous response. These may be part of an aberrant regeneration process (Fig. 22.4).

Midbrain corectopia

Damage to the third nerve fibres, even within the midbrain, may give rise to a sinuous pupil reaction. This has classically been described as an unequal upward and inward distortion of the pupil.

Episodic pupillary dysfunction ('springing pupil')

Episodic unilateral mydriasis lasting minutes to weeks and usually accompanied by blurred vision and headaches has been reported.

Spasms of the iris dilator giving rise to 'tadpole-shaped' pupils have been reported in young healthy adults. The pupils are peaked in one direction for a few minutes and this may occur on several separate occasions. This may represent a subset of patients with the springing pupil.

Paradoxical pupils

This is a curious phenomena in which the pupil size in the light is larger than in the dark. Although this was first reported to be pathognomonic for congenital stationary night blindness, it has been reported in association with cone disorders, Leber's amaurosis, dominant optic atrophy and even amblyopia. Nevertheless, in the young child with nystagmus, the presence of a paradoxical pupillary response suggests an electroretinogram should be obtained.

Horner's syndrome

Interruption of the sympathetic pathways subserving the eye is referred to as Horner's syndrome. Its characteristics include the following.

• *Miosis*. The pupillary responses to light and near stimulus in the affected eye is normal. The response to dark is slow and incomplete or absent.

• *Ptosis*. A 1–2-mm ptosis of the upper lid is present accompanied by a 1-mm elevation of the lower lid that gives the eyes an apparent enophthalmic appearance as the result of narrowing of the palpebral fissure.

• *Heterochromia*. Lighter pigmentation on the iris of the affected side occurs in some patients with congenital Horner's syndrome. It is not pathognomonic for a congenital Horner's syndrome and has been reported in patients with acquired causes (Fig. 22.5).

• *Anhidrosis*. Lesions prior to the superior cervical ganglion will interfere with sweating on the ipsilateral side of the face, resulting in a flushed face and conjunctiva, and nasal stuffiness.

Pharmacological testing may be done to confirm the diagnosis of Horner's syndrome although it is not usually necessary. The following tests may be performed.

1 Cocaine—will fail to dilate a Horner's pupil.

2 Hydroxyamphetamine — will dilate a first- or second-order neurone Horner's pupil but not a postganglionic one.

3 Adrenaline 0.1% — will not normally dilate the pupil but will in postganglionic Horner's syndrome with denervation hypersensitivity.

Horner's syndrome may be congenital or acquired. Congenital Horner's syndrome has been divided into three causal types.

1 With obstetrical trauma to the internal carotid and its sympathetic nerve plexus. These children were usually delivered by forceps and have the postganglionic Horner's syndrome.

2 With surgical or obstetrical trauma to the preganglionic sympathetic pathway. This group includes patients with brachial plexus injuries, known as Klumpke's palsy.

3 Those without a history of birth trauma but with a Horner's syndrome and evidence of a lesion at/or peripheral to the superior cervical ganglion. These patients have ipsilateral anhidrosis.

Acquired Horner's syndrome may likewise be characterized by their site or injury to the sympathetic pathway. These include the following.

1 A central lesion. This occurs with brainstem trauma, tumours, vascular malformations, infarcts, haemorrhages, syringomyelia and in comatose patients.

2 A preganglionic lesion. This occurs with neck trauma, neuroblastoma and other tumours in the area of the neck.

3 As a postganglionic neurone after the superior cervical ganglion. Lesions that account for this include cavernous sinus lesions, neuroblastoma and trauma.

Most Horner's syndromes seen in young children are congenital in nature. However, the occurrence of tumours in children with congenital Horner's syndrome has been reported. Thus, in some cases of congenital as well as acquired Horner's syndrome, investigations with a chest X-ray, head and neck tomogram and 24-hour catecholamine assay (evaluating for the presence of neuroblastoma) may be indicated (Fig. 22.6).

Lesions of the parasympathetics

In most cases of peripheral third nerve dysfunction, pupillary abnormalities are associated with signs of

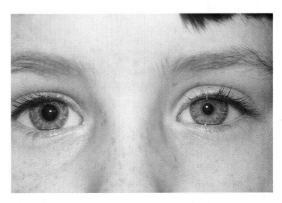

Fig. 22.6 Left Horner's syndrome. This child presented with the complaint of a sudden-onset ptosis and small pupil. Chest X-rays showed a left apical mass. The cause was a large benign ganglion neuroma; difficult to treat. In Horner's syndrome the pupil size difference is greater in the dark and the affected pupil is slower to dilate.

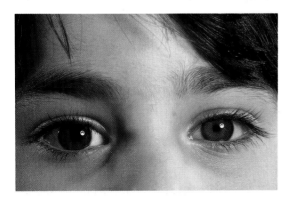

Fig. 22.5 Left congenital Horner's syndrome with heterochromia.

extraocular muscle and lid dysfunction. Occasionally, however, isolated internal ophthalmoplegia may occur as the result of a third nerve palsy. This usually results from selective compression of the pupillary motor fibres which are peripherally located in the nerve. In uncal herniation the comatose patient may develop a dilated pupil without evidence of extraocular muscle involvement for a period of some hours. However, if the condition continues to worsen ipsilateral external ophthalmoplegia and hemiplegia will invariably occur.

Pharmacological agents

Numerous pharmacological agents affect pupil size and reactivity. These agents may be applied topically to the eye or may be administered systemically.

Pupil-dilating agents
Parasympatholytic agents
These agents dilate the pupil and cause cycloplegia. They may cause respiratory failure in children with congenital central hypoventilation or seizures in the brain-damaged child. Commonly used agents are:
- atropine 0.5–1%;
- homatropine 2%;
- cyclopentolate 0.5–1%;
- tropicamide 1%;
- hyoscine 0.5%.

Sympathomimetics
These agents cause mild dilatation of the pupil and have no effect on accommodation. They must be used with great care and at a low dilution in premature babies since they have a pronounced effect on blood pressure and pulse rate. These agents include:
- adrenaline 0.1–1%;
- phenylephrine 2.5–10%.

Pupil-constricting agents
Cholinergic drugs
Pilocarpine 1–4% is commonly used to constrict the pupil as a treatment for glaucoma. It has little efficacy in the treatment of infantile glaucoma.

Anticholinesterases
These agents may be used to treat glaucoma or accommodative esotropia. They include:
- phospholine iodide (Ecothiopate) 0.03–0.125%;
- eserine 0.5%;
- isofluorophate 0.025%.

Sympatholytic agents
These include:
- guanethidine (Ismelin) 5%—occasionally used to treat lid retraction in hyperthyroidism;
- thymoxamine 1%.

Systemic agents
Atropine, scopolamine and benztropine can cause pupillary dilatation and accommodative paralysis when ingested in sufficient quantities. The seeds of the jimson weed, the berries of deadly nightshade and henbane have been known to cause a serious fatal poisoning. Mydriasis from topical atropine or atropine-like drugs is not counteracted by pilocarpine 1%, but in systemic poisoning it may be.

Antihistamines and some antidepressants produce mydriasis.

Heroin, morphine and other opiates, marijuana and some other psychotropic drugs cause bilateral pupil constriction.

Abnormalities of the near reflex

Congenital absence
Children may be born with a defect in the near reflex. They show no accommodation and poor convergence and the pupil fails to constrict to a near stimulus but constricts to light. The cause is unknown but may be peripheral in origin in a ciliary body or lens.

Acquired defects
Sylvian aqueduct (Parinaud's) syndrome
Premature presbyopia is one of the signs of tumours encroaching on the dorsal midbrain, accompanied by more classic signs of convergence–retraction nystagmus, vertical gaze defects, eyelid retraction, convergence defect and pupil light–near dissociation.

Systemic disease

Botulism, diphtheria, diabetes, head and neck trauma may all give rise to accommodative defects either in isolation or in association with eye movement and vergence defects. A defect in the near response has been reported in Wilson's disease.

Eye disease

Defective accommodation occurs in children with severe iridocyclitis, dislocated lenses, large colobomas, buphthalmos, very high myopia and direct eye trauma, including retinal detachment surgery.

Other neurological causes

Adie's tonic pupil syndrome and third nerve paralysis may cause defective accommodation.

Pharmacological agents

See above.

Psychogenic

Children in the second decade may present with symptoms of difficulty with reading due to non-organic causes. They can usually be cajoled into normal near responses or tricked by prisms and minus lenses.

Accommodation in school children

Although normal children have normal high amplitudes of accommodation, a small proportion have been reported to have abnormally low amplitudes. It is not clear if there is a statistical association with these low amplitudes of accommodation and learning disability.

Spasm of the near reflex

Spasm of the near reflex consists of episodes of a combination of accommodation-induced myopia, convergence of the eyes and miosis. The patient usually complains of blurred vision, double vision and ocular pain. This syndrome may be induced by overcorrecting myopic patients, but in most circumstances no organic disease can be found. The phenomena is assumed to be psychogenic. However, it has been described in association with:

- neurosyphilis;
- myasthenia gravis;
- multiple sclerosis;
- encephalitis.

Anisocoria

Anisocoria (unequal pupils) is seen frequently in a paediatric population and often causes unnecessary alarm. In most cases this is caused by physiological anisocoria.

Physiological anisocoria

This occurs in a significant proportion of the normal population. The resting size difference of the two pupils rarely exceeds 1 mm. The difference in size of the pupils remains apparent in bright light or in the dark. This is important in differentiating this condition from a Horner's syndrome or a parasympathetic lesion.

If the patient has a Horner's syndrome the pupillary size would be maximally different in the dark. If the patient has a lesion of the parasympathetic system the pupillary size will be of greatest disparity in bright light. If the patient has physiological anisocoria the difference in pupil size will remain the same, independent of the ambient lighting.

23: Leukaemia and the Eye

Leukaemia

Every part of the eye may be involved in leukaemia, especially now that the survival rates have greatly improved, and thus end-stage leukaemia is not so frequently encountered. The paediatric ophthalmologist less frequently sees patients with ocular complications. Nonetheless, they are important because they may cause considerable damage to one or both eyes and there may be signs of relapse or failure to respond to treatment.

Orbit
• Bone infiltration (Fig. 23.1) may occur with myeloid leukaemia. This is known as a chloroma.
• Soft tissue involvement occurs with lymphatic leukaemia in relapse.

Conjunctiva
Conjunctival infiltration occurs and haemorrhage may be related to the infiltration, hyperviscosity or coagulation defects.

Cornea and sclera
The cornea is rarely involved except by an associated herpes simplex or zoster infection in the immune compromised child.

Lens
Cataracts occur after bone marrow transplantation and total body irradiation.

Anterior chamber and iris
Iris relapse is an occasional site of extramedullary relapse, most frequently in lymphoblastic leukaemia after remission has been induced and treatment stopped but for 2 or 3 weeks. Iris relapse presents as:
• an isolated mass;
• sluggish pupil (Fig. 23.2);
• difference in colour between the two eyes;
• symptoms and signs of iritis;
• hyphaema;
• glaucoma.

Diagnosis may require iris biopsy and anterior chamber tap, and treatment is by radiotherapy, usually 3000 cGy and topical steroid treatment.

Choroid
The choroid is the most frequently involved part of the eye in all types of leukaemia. It is rarely clinically apparent but may present as a retinal detachment or subretinal mass.

Retinal and vitreous changes
1 Hyperviscosity giving rise to tortuous and dilated retinal veins, sheathing and haemorrhages (Fig. 23.3).
2 Retinal haemorrhages:
   (a) white centred haemorrhages due to leukaemic deposits with rupture of vessels (Fig. 23.4);
   (b) subhyaloid haemorrhages (Fig. 23.5);
   (c) nerve fibre layer and other haemorrhages also occur.
3 White retinal patches:
   (a) vessel sheathing;
   (b) retinal infiltrates, often haemorrhagic;
   (c) cotton wool spots — these occur most frequently after bone marrow transplantation (Fig. 23.6);
   (d) hard exudates related to leaking vessels;
   (e) white patches related to opportunistic cytomegalovirus or fungal infections;
   (f) retinal infarction giving rise to large areas of cloudy swelling of retinal nerve fibres.

Optic nerve involvement
• Common as a preterminal event.

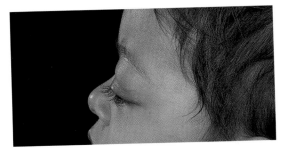

Fig. 23.1 Myeloid leukaemia presenting as proptosis and orbital mass ('chloroma').

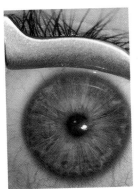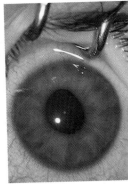

Fig. 23.2 Iris relapse with heterochromia, infiltrated iris and sluggish pupil reactions.

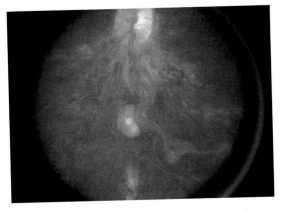

Fig. 23.3 Hyperviscosity changes in chronic myeloid leukaemia in a 20 year old.

- More rare recently.
- Loss of central vision.
- Prelamina infiltration shows swollen optic disc.
- Retrolamina infiltration detectable by scanning only.

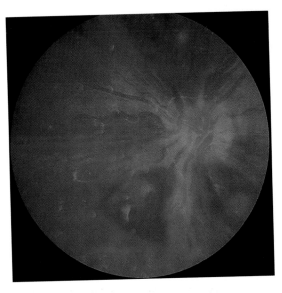

Fig. 23.4 White-centred and nerve fibre retinal haemorrhages in acute lymphatic leukaemia. There are several subhyaloid haemorrhages around the optic disc.

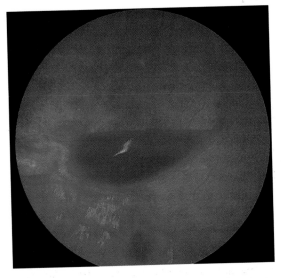

Fig. 23.5 Subhyaloid haemorrhages with acute lymphatic leukaemia associated with profound anaemia and thrombocytopenia.

Complications of treatment

Drugs

- Vincristine:
  (a) optic neuropathy;

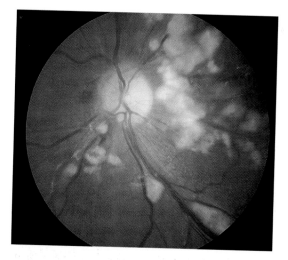

Fig. 23.6 Transient multiple cotton wool spots after bone marrow transplantation.

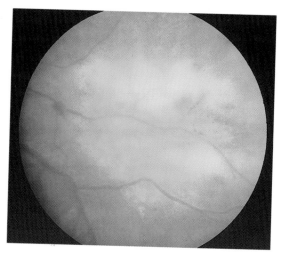

Fig. 23.8 Cytomegalovirus retinitis in acute lymphatic leukaemia in relapse.

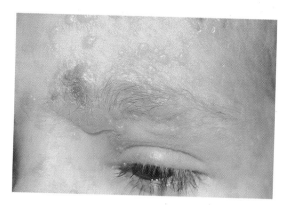

Fig. 23.7 Confluent varicella in a patient with acute lymphatic leukaemia in relapse.

  (b) ptosis;
  (c) cranial nerve palsy.
• L-asparaginase—encephalopathy.
• Cytarabine—corneal and conjunctival inflammation.
• Methotrexate—arachnoiditis.

• Steroids:
  (a) cataracts;
  (b) benign intracranial hypertension.

Immunosuppression

Opportunistic bacterial, viral, fungal or protozoal infections, i.e. herpes zoster (Fig. 23.7) or cytomegalovirus (Fig. 23.8).

Complications of bone marrow transplantation

1 Cataracts.
2 Transient retinal white spots.
3 Graft versus host disease:
  (a) failure to recognize the transplant recipient as 'self';
  (b) dry eye;
  (c) cicatricial lagophthalmos;
  (d) sterile conjunctivitis;
  (e) uveitis;
  (f) cataract.

24: The Phakomatoses

The phakomatoses (sometimes referred to as neuro-cutaneous disorders) are a group of syndromes in which skin, eye and central nervous system may be involved with benign tissue overgrowth. Included in this group is neurofibromatosis, tuberous sclerosis, von Hippel–Lindau disease and the Sturge–Weber syndrome.

Neurofibromatosis

Neurofibromatosis includes at least two clinically distinct autosomal dominant forms: (i) neuro-fibromatosis type 1 (NF1), von Recklinghausen's syndrome; and (ii) NF2, bilateral acoustic neurofibromatosis. Additional forms of neurofibromatosis have been described, including segmental neurofibromatosis, cutaneous NF3 mixed, NF4 variant and NF7 late onset. It is not certain that all of these forms represent distinct separate disease entities.

NF1
Diagnostic criteria
The following have been defined as the criteria for establishing the diagnosis of NF1. At least two must be present in order to establish the diagnosis.
1 Five or more café au lait spots over 5 mm in diameter in pre-pubertal patients and six or more café au lait spots over 15 mm in diameter in post-pubertal patients.
2 Two or more neurofibromas of any type or one plexiform neurofibroma.
3 Axillary or inguinal freckling.
4 Optic glioma.
5 Two or more Lisch nodules.
6 A distinctive osseous lesion (pseudoarthrosis of the tibia or sphenoid wing dysplasia) (Fig. 24.1).
7 A first-degree relative with NF1.

Prevalence
The prevalence of neurofibromatosis has been estimated to be 1:3000–1:5000 making it one of the most common autosomal dominant conditions in humans. Penetrance is nearly complete but a high spontaneous mutation rate results in nearly 50% of the patients diagnosed representing new mutations. The involved gene has been isolated to the proximal long arm of chromosome 17 (17q11.2).

Systemic features
• Café au lait spots and freckling. Café au lait spots are not pathognomonic of neurofibromatosis and may occur in normal subjects.
• Freckling in skin creases occurs in the axilla, inguinal region and submammary folds in women.

Peripheral neurofibromas
Nearly all patients with NF1 develop cutaneous peripheral neurofibromas by the age of 16 years. Less commonly seen are subcutaneous peripheral neurofibromas palpable along peripheral nerves.

Plexiform neurofibromas
These are ill-defined tumours which are soft on palpation. They are pathognomonic of NF1. Hypertrophy of the surrounding tissues with regional overgrowth and hypertrichosis in the involved area are common features. When they involve the orbit significant visual impairment may result as a direct result of compression of the optic nerve or from the amblyopia resulting from the ptosis and/or strabismus created by the tumour.

Cognitive impairment
Mental retardation is rare in NF1 but a mild visual perceptual difficulty has been reported.

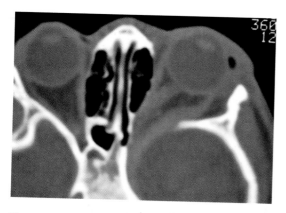

Fig. 24.1 NF1. Computerized tomography scan showing bony sphenoid defect.

Ophthalmological features

Ophthalmological assessment of patients with suspected NF1 is important not only to confirm the diagnosis but also to detect the ophthalmic complications and to institute treatment as early as possible. Ophthalmological involvement may occur in the orbit. Orbital involvement may be due to:

1 optic nerve glioma;
2 optic nerve sheath meningioma;
3 orbital neurofibroma;
4 defects of the orbital bones.

Proptosis may be associated with displacement of the globe with resulting strabismus and amblyopia. Tumours in the orbit frequently cause optic nerve changes with papilloedema, optic atrophy and, occasionally, optic nerve hypoplasia. Additional findings include:

1 optociliary shunts (particularly with optic nerve sheath meningiomas);
2 choroidal folds;
3 gaze-evoked amaurosis.

Neuroimaging studies are indicated to differentiate between the various causes of proptosis in NF1.

The eyelids

1 Eyelid involvement may occur as the result of plexiform neurofibromas, often causing a characteristic 'S'-shaped deformity of the upper lid margin. Strabismus and/or ptosis resulting from this involvement may lead to amblyopia.

2 Congenital ptosis may be present even in the absence of orbital tumours.

Iris

Lisch nodules (melanocytic hamartomas of the iris) are specific for NF1. They are rarely seen in NF2. The prevalence of Lisch nodules in NF1 increases with age. They are infrequently seen in infancy but are found in nearly 100% of patients with neurofibromatosis by the age of 20 years.

Optic nerve

Optic nerve involvement is primarily involved with optic nerve gliomas (pilocytic astrocytomas) (Fig. 24.2). Seventy per cent of all optic gliomas occur in patients with NF1. The true prevalence rate in NF1 is difficult as many remain asymptomatic and thus subclinical. As many as 15% of patient with NF1 and normal visual acuity have been found to have radiographic evidence of optic nerve gliomas. Gliomas of the optic nerve may be divided into two categories.

Anterior (orbital)

These gliomas present with proptosis, visual loss and occasional subluxation of the globe. Involvement of the optic nerve may occur as atrophy, dysplasia, direct tumour involvement or swelling. Optociliary shunt vessels occasionally occur on the side of the tumour. Strabismus commonly results.

Posterior (chiasmal gliomas)

(See Chapter 19.) These gliomas present with hydrocephalus, endocrine abnormalities or visual impairment associated with nystagmus. The nystagmus may be vertical, rotatory or asymmetrical (occasionally mimicking spasmus nutans). See-saw nystagmus is frequently seen.

The conjunctiva

Neurofibromas of the conjunctiva are rare and tend to affect the limbal area.

Cornea

Thickening of the corneal nerves may occur in NF1 but is not pathognomonic for it. It is seen much more commonly in the multiple endocrine neoplasia syndrome.

Uveal tract

Pigmentory hamartomas of the choroid may be seen in up to 35% of patients. Diffuse neurofibromas may cause thickening of the entire uveal tract, resulting in glaucoma.

Retina

Involvement of the retina in NF1 is rare. Occasional cases have been reported of retinal astrocytic hamartomas and combined hamartomas of the retina and retinal pigment epithelium.

Investigations

1 Computerized tomography (CT) or magnetic resonance imaging (MRI) of the brain and orbits. These are important in detecting bony abnormalities, meningioma or optic nerve glioma.
2 Visual evoked potentials (VEPs) may be useful in monitoring progression or regression of chiasmal gliomas or in assessing chiasmal involvement.

Management

Management of patients with NF1 is often complex and controversial. Genetic counselling should be an essential part in the management of all family members of an affected patient. Treatment of the ocular complications of neurofibromatosis is difficult. It may include the following.

Plexiform neuroma

This is not sensitive to chemotherapy or radiotherapy. Surgical resection is difficult with a significant complication rate. Occlusion therapy may be necessary if amblyopia is suspected.

Optic nerve and chiasmal gliomas

Treatment remains controversial. Conservative treatment is indicated if little or no visual loss is detected. Radiation therapy may be indicated occasionally in the older patient (mental retardation will occur if radiation is used in the young child). Surgical resection may be indicated with marked proptosis and a blind eye. Surgical removal of chiasmal gliomas is not technically possible. Occasionally a

cystic component may be removed. Chemotherapy is becoming more popular in the treatment of chiasmal gliomas associated with hypothalamic dysfunction. Shunting for raised intracranial pressure may be necessary in some patients with chiasmal gliomas. Endocrinological evaluation of patients with chiasmal gliomas is important.

Glaucoma

This usually requires surgery and even then prognosis is poor.

NF2 (bilateral acoustic) (Fig. 24.2)

This form is much less common than NF1. The responsible gene has been located near the centre of the long arm of chromosome 22 (22q11.1–q13.1).

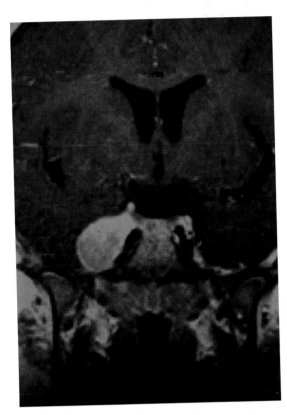

Fig. 24.2 NF2. This 2-year-old boy with NF2 presented with a long-standing head tilt. An enhancing lesion, probably a meningioma, fills the cavernous sinus and floor of the middle cranial fossa.

Systemic features

- Café au lait spots—occur in approximately 60% of patients.
- Cutaneous neurofibromas—occur in approximately 30% of patients. Plexiform neuromas are rare.

Central nervous system features

The hallmark of neurofibromatosis is bilateral acoustic neuromas. Other cranial nerves may be involved with tumour growth, especially nerves V, VI and VII. Commonly, gliomas, meningiomas and schwannomas occur.

Ophthalmic features

- Lisch nodules rarely, if ever, occur.
- Posterior subcapsular lens opacities are common but are rarely visually significant.
- Combined pigment epithelial and retinal hamartomas.
- Epiretinal membranes with mild visual loss.

In most cases no treatment is indicated for the ophthalmological manifestations of NF2. Treatment is aimed at the bilateral VIIIth nerve meningiomas where surgical resection is usually preferred, particularly if the tumours are small.

Tuberous sclerosis

The triad of mental retardation, epilepsy and vesiculopapillar rash on the face in association with cerebral tumours is considered to be characteristic of tuberous sclerosis. Tuberous sclerosis is associated with multiple developmental tumours and is inherited as an autosomal dominant disorder. However, at least 75% of cases are spontaneous mutations. The complete syndrome has never been reported in two consecutive generations. At least two different gene loci have been associated with this disorder — chromosome 9 (9q34) and chromosome 11 (11q22–q23).

Diagnostic criteria

Diagnosis of tuberous sclerosis may be made when there is one primary feature or two secondary features.

Primary features

- Periungual fibroma (Fig. 24.3).
- Retinal hamartomas (more than one).
- Facial angiofibromas (Fig. 24.4).
- Subependymal glial nodules (on neuroimaging studies).
- Multiple cortical tubers (Fig. 24.5).
- Bilateral renal angiomyolipomas.

If an individual has an affected first-degree relative tuberous sclerosis may be diagnosed if one of the following is present:

- Shagreen patch;
- forehead fibrous plaque;
- multiple cardiac rhabdomyomas;
- giant cell astrocytoma;
- isolated retinal phakoma;
- isolated cortical tuber.

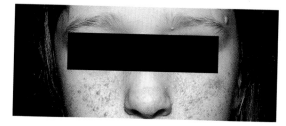

Fig. 24.3 Periungual fibromas.

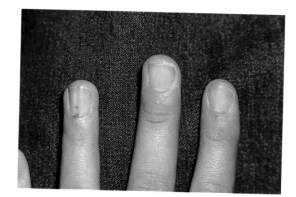

Fig. 24.4 Tuberous sclerosis, angiofibromas of the face—most characteristically seen, as here, over the malar region.

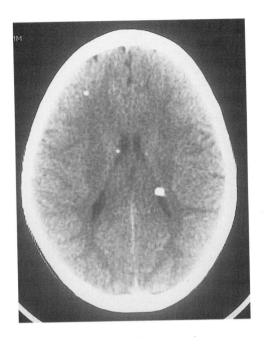

Fig. 24.5 Periventricular calcification in tuberous sclerosis.

Secondary features

If no first-degree relative is affected two of the following features in an individual are diagnostic of the condition:

- hypomelanotic macules;
- bilateral polycystic kidneys;
- isolated cardiac rhabdomyoma;
- isolated renal angiomyolipoma;
- pulmonary lymphangiomyomatosis;
- multiple cortical or subcortical hypomyelinated lesions.

Systemic features

Skin signs

Angiofibromas

These are rare before the age of 2 years but are present in 85% of affected individuals by adulthood. The lesions characteristically involve the butterfly distribution over the nose and cheeks, sparing the upper lip but involving the chin.

Hypomelanotic patches

These must commonly take the form of 'ash-leaf patches' and are clinically seen as a white patch with a long axis, usually in a line of a dermatome. They may be seen in the first year of life (a Wood's ultraviolet lamp may be required to detect them) but they are not pathognomonic for tuberous sclerosis.

Shagreen patches

In 40% of tuberous sclerosis patients these thickened patches of discoloured skin, usually involving the lumbar area, are seen (Fig. 24.6).

Forehead fibrous plaques

These may be present at birth and are pathognomonic of the condition but are only present in 25% of patients. They appear as raised red, waxy skin lesions.

Fibromas

Subungual and periungual fibromas may grow from the nails of hands or feet. Less commonly, fibromas of the gum are seen. Skin tags may occur on the back of the neck and shoulders. Fibromas occur in 50% of patients.

Visceral signs

Patients with tuberous sclerosis may have renal, cardiac, pulmonary and other visceral involvement.

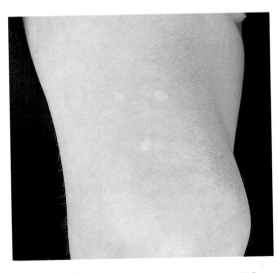

Fig. 24.6 Tuberous sclerosis. Ash-leaf spots are small flat depigmented areas on the skin which occur anywhere on the body, are usually lanceolate in shape and are best seen with a Woods ultraviolet light.

Renal

Multiple angiomyolipomas of the kidney or benign renal cysts.

Cardiac

Rhabdomyomas, usually multiple but rarely symptomatic.

Pulmonary

Subpleural cysts, pulmonary fibrosis with secondary emphysema.

Neurological involvement

- *Seizures*:
    (a) in infancy and early childhood — infantile spasms;
    (b) in older children—grand mal seizures.
- *Mental retardation* occurs in approximately 60% of patients.
- *Intracranial lesions.*
- *Cortical tubers* and *subependymal nodules*. These are both hamartomas and can be seen on CT or MRI. Occasional malignant transformation occurs and accounts for approximately 25% of premature deaths in tuberous sclerosis.

Ophthalmological features

The overwhelming, most common ophthalmic features in tuberous sclerosis are the retinal hamartomas and other abnormalities of the posterior pole.

Phakomas (retinal hamartomas)

These occur in approximately 50% of patients and are bilateral in at least 50% of affected patients. They may be flat, smooth and semi-transparent, or raised, calcific and a typical 'mulberry-like' tumour. Intermediate forms combining features of both may also be seen. These lesions are usually static and do not show significant growth (Fig. 24.7).

Retinal vascular anomalies

Those associated with the tumours include aneurysmal dilatation of vessels and primary arteriovenous malformations. These may lead to vitreous haemorrhage (Fig. 24.8).

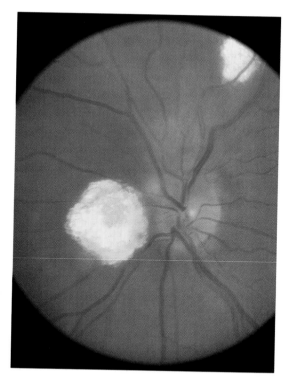

Fig. 24.7 Tuberous sclerosis. 'Mulberry tumours'—these white elevated refractive hamartomas probably evolved from flat translucent lesions.

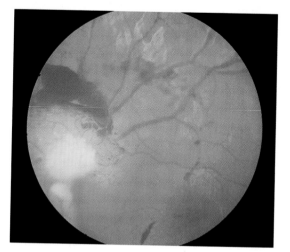

Fig. 24.8 Patient with tuberous sclerosis showing vitreous haemorrhage associated with a retinal hamartoma.

Pigmentory abnormalities

'Punch-out' depigmented areas in the midperiphery of the retina have been reported in this syndrome (Fig. 24.9).

Optic disc abnormalities

Swelling of the optic nerve head or optic atrophy may occur. Rarely, optic disc anomalies including tilted discs and colobomas may occur.

Non-retinal features

These other ocular features that have been reported in association with tuberous sclerosis include:

- megalocornea;
- keratoconus;
- posterior embryotoxon;
- glaucoma;
- cataract.

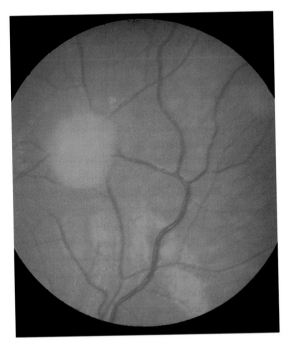

Fig. 24.9 Tuberous sclerosis. Almost flat translucent retinal lesions overlying blood vessels.

Sturge–Weber syndrome

The Sturge–Weber syndrome is a rare, neuro-oculocutaneous disorder. In its classic presentation it presents with a portwine stain affecting the skin supplied by the trigeminal nerve on one side of the face. The neurological manifestations are epilepsy, mental retardation and hemiplegia. The main ocular manifestation is glaucoma. The genetic mechanism that is responsible for this syndrome remains controversial. Most authorities consider it to be due to a somatic mutation during early development but others suggest that the disorder may be caused by a lethal gene surviving by mosaicism. The embryogenesis of the disorder most likely involves incomplete differentiation of the primordial vascular mesenchyme of the cephalic ectoderm and the underlying neural tube between 4 and 8 weeks gestational age. Alternatively, it has been suggested that the defect is a result of failure of cortical veins to connect with the superior sagittal sinus resulting in a leptomeningeal vascular malformation that represents collateral circulation.

Diagnostic criteria

Complete trisymptomatic Sturge–Weber syndrome

- Neurocutaneous angiomatosis.
- Leptomeningeal angiomatosis (Fig. 24.10).
- Ocular involvement.
- Cutaneous angiomatosis.

Incomplete bisymptomatic Sturge–Weber syndrome (Fig. 24.11)

- Oculocutaneous angiomatosis.
- Neurocutaneous angiomatosis.

Incomplete monosymptomatic Sturge–Weber syndrome

- Isolated leptomeningeal angiomatosis.
- Isolated trigeminal cutaneous angiomatosis.

Extended Sturge–Weber syndrome

Those cases associated with other neurocutaneous syndromes including:

- Klippel–Trenaunay–Weber syndrome;
- oculodermal melanosis (naevus of Ota);

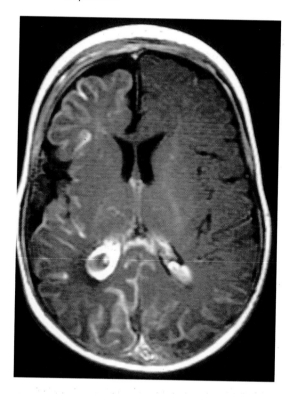

Fig. 24.10 Sturge–Weber syndrome showing hemicerebral atrophy and calcification.

- neurofibromatosis;
- tuberous sclerosis;
- von Hippel–Lindau disease;
- Wyburn–Mason syndrome;
- cutis marmorata telangiectatica congenita;
- neurocutaneous melanosis;
- phakomatosis pigmentovascularis type IVa.

von Hippel–Lindau disease

Angiomatosis of the retina and cerebellum constitutes the syndrome known as the von Hippel–Lindau disorder (Fig. 24.12). The disorder is inherited as autosomal dominant and a gene has been identified on the short arm of chromosome 3 (3p25–p26). The major features of this disorder include retinal angiomatosis, cerebellar/medullar and spinal cord haemangioblastomas (Fig. 24.13), renal cell carcinoma and phaeochromocytoma.

Clinical variability is common in these patients and rarely are all features present in any given patient.

Systemic manifestations
Neurological
Lesions of the central nervous system are almost always below the tentorium. The most common is cerebellar haemangioblastoma, occurring in about 20% of patients. Similar lesions may affect the

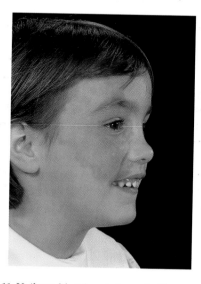

Fig. 24.11 Unilateral facial portwine stain. The patient is in the early stages of having laser treatment for the portwine stain.

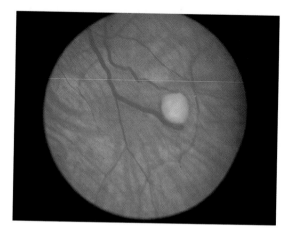

Fig. 24.12 von Hippel–Lindau syndrome. Haemangioblastoma with large feeding and draining vessel.

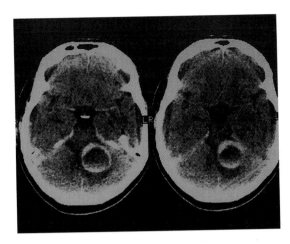

Fig. 24.13 von Hippel–Lindau syndrome showing cerebellar haemangioblastoma.

medullar and spinal cord less commonly. Syringobulbae and syringomyelia may also occur.

Visceral
The kidney may be affected by clear-cell carcinoma or haemangioblastoma. Less commonly, haemangioma may affect the pancreas. Phaeochromocytomas occur in about 10% of patients. Paraganglioma of the epididymis is uncommon.

Ophthalmic manifestations
Retinal angiomatosis occurs in about two-thirds of cases. These are usually located in the midperiphery and five stages of development of these lesions have been described.
- *Stage 1.* Pre-classical; small capillary clusters, initially only the size of diabetic microaneurysms.
- *Stage 2.* Classical; typical retinal angiomas.
- *Stage 3.* Exudation; from leaking vessels of the tumour.
- *Stage 4.* Retinal detachment; exudative or tractual.
- *Stage 5.* End-stage; retinal detachment, uveitis, glaucoma, phthisis.

Early treatment of the retinal lesions is indicated and will be associated with less complications. Cryotherapy, laser therapy, surgical resection and radiation therapy have all been utilised.

Those affected with von Hippel–Lindau should be screened with the following examinations:
1 annual medical history and physical examination;
2 ophthalmological examination every 6–12 months from age 6 years;
3 urine test for phaeochromocytoma at least once, and if blood pressure becomes elevated or unstable it should be repeated;
4 bilateral selective renal angiography after age 15–20 years, repeated every 1–5 years;
5 MRI of the posterior fossa;
6 CT scan of the pancreas and kidney after age 15–20 years, repeated every 1–5 years or whenever symptoms occur.

It has also been suggested that children of affected parents and/or other close relatives at high risk should be screened in the following manner:
1 medical history of physical examination from age 10 years;
2 ophthalmological examination annually after age 6 years or if any suspicious signs occur;
3 urine testing for phaeochromocytoma at least once and, if blood pressure becomes elevated or unstable, repeated;
4 MRI of the posterior fossa and CT of the pancreas and kidneys at least once a decade after age 20 years;
5 pancreatic and renal sonography from age 15–20 years;
6 when available, family DNA studies should be done to determine who does or does not have the causative gene.

25: Trauma

Accidental trauma

Serious eye injuries in children in developed countries occur at a rate of about 12 per 100 000 head of population per year. Although usually unilateral, the consequences can be overwhelming if there is injury to or disease of the other eye at a later date. The cosmetic significance can be large and employment prospects are reduced by the trauma. Younger children, especially boys, are more at risk and injuries tend to occur more frequently in socially deprived circumstances where parental supervision and education is lacking.

Eyelid trauma

This occurs either associated with facial trauma or it may be isolated, in the case of a dog or another animal bite, when canalicular injuries are frequent.

Canalicular injuries require intubation via the intact canaliculus, suturing the wound with a synthetic tube left in place. Common canalicular injuries require microdissection and intubation of the nasolacrimal system via both upper and lower canaliculi.

Subconjunctival haemorrhages

(See Chapter 10.) It is important to remember that subconjunctival haemorrhage may mask an underlying penetrating injury, perforating injury or eye wall trauma. The haemorrhage itself clears rapidly without treatment.

Corneal abrasions

Corneal abrasions occur when the cornea is scraped with a blunt object such as a nail, stick, etc. The abrasion is assessed with fluorescein drops and foreign material removed. The eye is usually patched, with antibiotic ointment instilled in the eye and analgesics. Cycloplegia may help to avoid ciliary spasm.

Eye wall laceration

This mostly affects the cornea to the limbus and sometimes the anterior sclera (Fig. 25.1). Almost invariably there is damage to the intraocular contents, except when the penetration is by a very small object, i.e. a needle.

Investigations
1 The other eye must be examined, including dilated ophthalmoscopy.
2 Slit lamp examination is mandatory to assess the extent of the damage as far as can be seen (details may be obscured by haemorrhage).
3 Intraocular pressure must be measured if possible. If full-thickness laceration has occurred the pressure will be low.
4 Ultrasound examination is useful, especially when there is anterior segment haemorrhage or cataract, to assess whether the posterior segment is involved and to help exclude intraocular foreign body. Computerised tomography (CT) scanning examination is helpful to exclude intraocular foreign body, orbital foreign body, fractures and retrobulbar haemorrhage. Magnetic resonance imaging (MRI) should not be performed if a metallic foreign body is suspected.

Management
Nearly all small children require anaesthetic and, if the laceration is full thickness, anaesthetic is required except for very small lesions. Anaesthesia is induced, usually avoiding a depolarising muscle relaxant. The wound, either corneoscleral or corneal scleral, is closed using fine absorbable or non-absorbable sutures. Non-absorbable corneal sutures

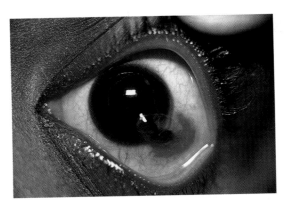

Fig. 25.1 Penetrating injury with iris prolapse and subconjunctival haemorrhage. (Photograph courtesy of Dr William Good.)

usually need to be removed early with children, especially once they become loose. Any hyphaema is washed out simultaneously if:

1 there is severe lens damage and incipient cataract formation, lensectomy is performed immediately and if the posterior capsule is intact an intraocular lens may be placed at the time of primary surgery or later; and

2 if there is posterior segment damage with a vitreous haemorrhage, concurrent vitrectomy or retinal surgery may be appropriate.

Penetrating and perforating injuries

The management of these is the same as lacerations except that there is a foreign body involved; intraocular in the case of penetrating injuries and in perforating injuries the foreign body has passed right through the eye. The difference in management from eye wall lacerations depends on the nature of the foreign body. Most intraocular foreign bodies require removal: this is usually accomplished by the use of intraocular microsurgical forceps. Iron foreign bodies have been removed by the use of a giant magnet but microsurgery makes this rarely necessary. Non-toxic orbital foreign bodies rarely need to be removed and sometimes small glass or Perspex intraocular foreign bodies may be left but, as a general rule, it is best to remove all foreign material.

> **Box 25.1 Hyphaema in childhood**
>
> *Causes*
> - Trauma—accidental or non-accidental.
> - Tumours:
>   (a) juvenile xanthogranuloma;
>   (b) leukaemia;
>   (c) Langerhan's cell histiocytosis;
>   (d) medulloepithelioma;
>   (e) retinoblastoma.
> - Rubeosis:
>   (a) retinal dysplasia;
>   (b) persistent hyperplastic vitreous (PHPV);
>   (c) retinopathy of prematurity (ROP);
>   (d) sickle cell anaemia.
> - Iris vascular malformation.
> - Iridoschisis.
> - Iritis and iris rubeosis.
> - Blood coagulation disorders, scurvy, purpura.
> - PHPV.
> - Iris melanoma.
>
> *Management*
> 1 Immediate—rule out other intraocular damage.
> 2 Rest—as far as is possible with a small child!
> 3 Watch the intraocular pressure.
> 4 Avoid aspirin or non-steroidal anti-inflammatories.
> 5 Wash out anterior chamber only if the hyphaema fails to spontaneously resolve after, say, 3 days or if there is severely raised intraocular pressure.
>
> *Long-term management*
> Rule out angle recession, dislocated lens, posterior segment damage. If there is angle recession these patients are usually followed for life because of the possible development of glaucoma.

Blunt injury

Blunt injuries may cause a number of intraocular problems.

1 Hyphaema.
2 Lens dislocation and cataract.
3 Iris damage and angle recession.
4 Retinal damage.
   (a) Commotio retinae:
      (i) white retinal sheen due to retinal oedema;
      (ii) if macular involved the vision is poor;
      (iii) generally good prognosis;
      (iv) sometimes permanent central vision loss;

(v) lamellar or full-thickness macular hole may result.

(b) Choroidal rupture (see below).

(c) Purtscher's:

(i) trauma associated with raised central venous pressure;

(ii) similar appearance in fat or air embolism;

(iii) widespread retinal infarcts and haemorrhage;

(iv) visual prognosis variable.

(d) Retinal haemorrhages:

(i) all retinal layers especially subhyaloid;

(ii) suggests other intraocular injuries;

(iii) associated with retinal breaks.

(e) Retinal detachment—occurs even with retinal breaks.

Scleral rupture

Rupture occurs when the sclera splits due to a non-penetrating injury which often occurs around the optic disc: the eye contents are forced out. Anterior ruptures are usually associated with eye wall laceration. Causes include small balls such as squash balls, fists, sticks, etc.

• Any blunt injury carries the risk of rupture.

• Intraocular pressure is low.

• Ultrasound shows vitreous haemorrhage and sometimes posterior bowing of the sclera. CT may show orbital haemorrhage.

• Blow-out fractures may accompany the rupture.

Anterior ruptures can be treated surgically, as with eye wall lacerations. Posterior ruptures are usually beyond repair.

Prevention of eye injuries

• Improvement of parental supervision. Supervision at school, playgroups, etc.

• Parental education about the dangers of eye injuries, and the times at which they occur.

• The use of protective goggles, especially for the one-eyed person, in a situation where the eye is in danger, i.e. small ball sports, metal on metal and metal on stone occupations, etc.

Orbital trauma

Blunt injuries to the orbital wall may cause fractures with or without displacement. Displaced fractures usually require treatment, undisplaced fractures do not.

Complications

• Brown's syndrome.

• Large posterior fractures may give rise to enophthalmos.

• Blow-out fracture:

(a) rare in early childhood;

(b) inferior or medial wall fracture with entrapment of orbital contents;

(c) enophthalmos;

(d) hypotropic eye or other primary position deviation;

(e) vertical, especially upwards, movements defective;

(f) concomitant intraocular ocular injury;

(g) treatment

(i) minor degrees of blow-out fractures require no treatment when there is marked enophthalmos and severely limited movements

(ii) orbital floor replacement with a Silastic or other synthetic implant may be helpful.

Cranial nerve injuries

Third, fourth and sixth nerve palsies are frequent in head injuries. Usually no treatment is necessary because many recover. Sometimes, especially with sixth nerve palsies, botulinum toxin into the ipsilateral antagonist may be helpful in the acute phase. Generally, the double vision is managed by patching or prisms, and at least 6 months is left after stabilisation of the deviation before any surgery. Patching should be done over the non-paretic eye in an attempt to keep the paretic eye moving and thus avoid further rectus muscle contracture.

Traumatic optic neuropathy

May occur by avulsion, from the globe, involvement in the fracture or ischaemic damage resulting from damage to the blood supply or an optic nerve sheath haemorrhage. Diagnosis is by ultrasound or neuroimaging, pupil signs and fundus examination. High-dose steroids or optic canal decompression may be helpful in appropriate cases.

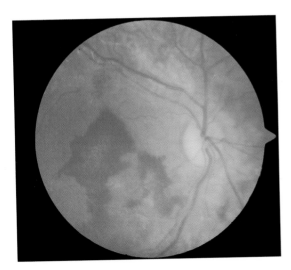

Fig. 25.2 Intraretinal, subretinal and subhyaloid haemorrhages in non-accidental injury.

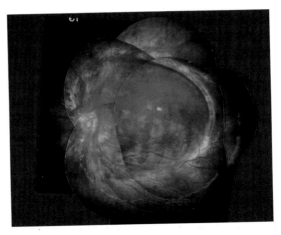

Fig. 25.4 Perimacular retinal folds. The raised nature of the folds can be seen by the shadow created by the fold above. Perimacular folds are suggestive, but not pathognomonic, of non-accidental injury.

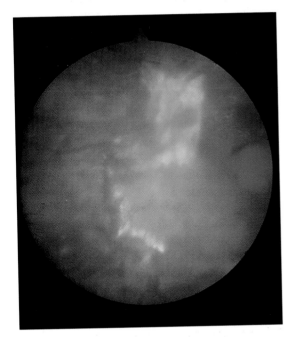

Fig. 25.3 Retinal and vitreous haemorrhages in non-accidental injury. The white areas represent partially organized haemorrhage and the greenish background is caused by altered blood products. Bright red haemorrhages are likely to be more recent than organized haemorrhages.

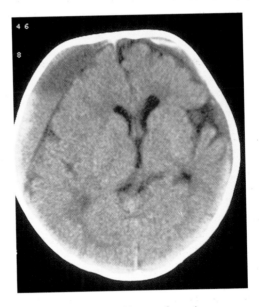

Fig. 25.5 Bilateral subdural haemorrhages in a non-accidentally injured child.

Non-accidental trauma

- Increasingly frequently diagnosed.
- Serious emotional and other sequelae.
- Mostly very young children.
- A variety of mechanisms, frequently shaking injuries.
- Poor psychosocial background—younger parents—stressing social or work situation—history of other forms of abuse, i.e. spouse abuse, personal violence, etc.—abuser was often abused.

Ocular complications
Retinal haemorrhages
Retinal haemorrhages are not pathognomonic of non-accidental injury, but widespread retinal haemorrhages occur much more frequently and are more severe in non-accidental than in accidental haemorrhage. There are two mechanisms for retinal haemorrhage:
1 rise in intravenous and intraocular pressure;
2 shaking with rapid acceleration and deceleration.
   All types of haemorrhages occur, for example:
1 vitreous haemorrhage—preretinal;
2 subhyaloid haemorrhage (Fig. 25.2);
3 haemorrhages of varying ages (Fig. 25.3);
4 perimacular folds with retinal haemorrhages (Fig. 25.4)—these are elevated folds in the retina and choroid in the arcuate area related to shaking injury (usually, but not necessarily, non-accidental);
5 haemorrhages in any other retinal layer (Fig. 25.5).

Central nervous system injury
The severity of the eye injury reflects the severity of intracranial damage probably because the mechanisms are similar. Hemispherical haemorrhage and subdural haematomas (Fig. 25.5) are frequent.

Other ocular injuries
- Periocular bruising.
- Cataract.
- Dislocated lenses.
- Traumatic mydriasis.
- Cigarette burns on cheek or lids (especially more than one).
- Retinal detachment.
- Intralamellar retinoschisis.

See D. Taylor (ed.), Chapters 62 and P29, *Paediatric Ophthalmology*, 2nd edn, 1997, Blackwell Science, Oxford.

Box 25.2 Management of suspected non-accidental injury

1 Admit to hospital.
2 Collaborate with paediatricians, etc.
3 Full history and examination, preferably with photographs.
4 Full documentation.
5 Involvement of social services.
6 Search for other injury, X-ray, CT, MRI, bone scan, etc.
7 Exclude bleeding diathesis.
8 Ongoing liaison with parents and agencies.
9 Police informed when diagnosis definite.
10 Protocols differ regionally.

The doctor must maintain a fair, non-vindictive, non-superior and helpful attitude towards the family at all times.

Box 25.3 Differential diagnosis of non-accidental injury

1 Osteogenesis imperfecta.
2 Bleeding diathesis; leukaemia.
3 Copper deficiency.
4 Scurvy.
5 Accidental injury.

26: Non-organic Visual Disorders

The nomenclature of these conditions is difficult. Names such as hysteria, functional or psychogenic disorder are sometimes unacceptable to parents and do not correctly reflect the underlying disorder. More correctly, conversion disorder or stress-related visual loss have been used. There is a distinct difference between these patients in whom the condition is unconscious and malingerers who feign visual loss.

Presentation

- Rare under 6 years old.
- Average age 10 years.
- Females three times more common than males.
- Family disharmony common.
- Family history of eye disease may be present.
- Patients often little inconvenienced by their condition.
- Vision often 'deteriorates' on subsequent examination.
- Symptoms usually of:
  (a) not seeing;
  (b) blurred vision;
  (c) distorted vision;
  (d) rarely, field defects or 'tunnel vision'.
- Other non-organic defects occasionally occur:
  (a) spasm of the near reflex;
  (b) headaches;
  (c) voluntary nystagmus;
  (d) others.

Clues in the history

The key to the diagnosis is from the history:
- sudden onset related to specific events or situations;
- step-like deterioration with each examination;
- patient little inconvenienced by their condition.

Psychological background

At home
- Sibling rivalry.
- Family disharmony.
- Teasing or bullying by neighbours.
- Overcrowding.
- Sexual abuse or harassment by relatives or others.

At school
- Overstretching.
- Understretching.
- Unsympathetic or aggressive teachers.
- Teasing or bullying.
- Sexual or non-sexual harassment by other pupils.

Clues in the examination

The diagnosis of a non-organic visual disorder relies upon the finding of positively non-organic signs, not just the failure to find any abnormality.
- *Bilateral total blindness*:
  (a) normal pupil reactions despite claimed bilateral blindness;
  (b) involuntary eye movements to a patient's image in a moving mirror despite complete blindness (Fig. 26.1);
  (c) reflex blinking to threat;
  (d) optokinetic nystagmus present.
- *Unilateral blindness*:
  (a) lens confusion (Fig. 26.2);
  (b) Worth's dots—the patient may see an appropriate number of dots in the Worth's test;
  (c) stereoacuity inappropriate to the unilateral visual defect.
- *Partial visual loss*:
  (a) better acuity or visual fields achieved by coaxing;

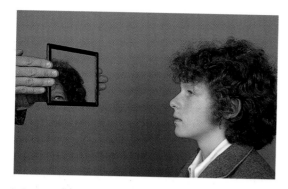

Fig. 26.1 When a blind person looks at a mirror, no movement takes place when the mirror is rotated. The sighted person's eyes will move as the mirror rotates, although he or she feels they are looking straightahead.

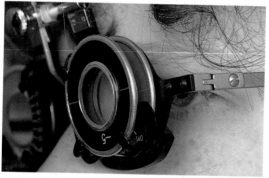

(a)

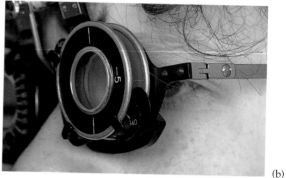

(b)

Fig. 26.2 The right eye is suspected of seeing better than the patient indicates; the ophthalmologist puts two cancelling cylinders at the same axis in front of the left eye (a), obscures the patient's view of the test type by moving across him, switches the lenses to add to each other (b) and occludes the left eye and, as he moves away from the patient, urges him to read quickly. The left eye is now obscured by the lens combination and the right eye is forced to be used. The patient does not usually detect the change of being forced to use the right eye.

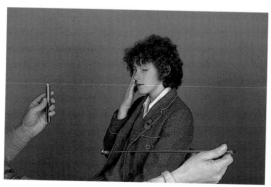

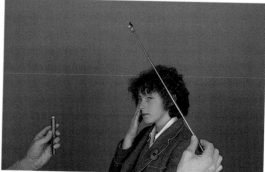

Fig. 26.3 The patient who has been shown to have very constricted visual fields on confrontation or other testing, looks accurately between the light and the mobile target which moves in the apparently blind part of the field. She is instructed to look at the torchlight and then to fix the peripheral target. When she has fixed the peripheral target she is told to look back to the torchlight, the peripheral target is moved in her apparently blind field and she is told to look back at it. This cannot be anything other than a non-organic defect providing that peripheral field constriction has been convincingly demonstrated beforehand.

(b) a monotonous and excessively slow reading of all letters, even the largest;

(c) acuities greatly differ in terms of angles subtended at different distances;

(d) high level of stereoacuity despite severely reduced visual acuity;

(e) normal prism tests despite severely reduced vision.

- *Visual field defects*:

(a) Tunnel vision, i.e. a visual field that is the same size at different distances. It is important to make sure that the distance difference is gross.

(b) Pilling of isoptres or isoptres pile at the same point. This can be organic. Accurate saccades into an apparently blind area (Fig. 26.3).

(c) Spiralling of visual fields. The fields become smaller as the test progresses.

Very few of the tests are absolutely pathognomonic. The diagnosis mainly relies on the demonstration of clearly non-organic visual field defects, especially abnormal saccading into an apparently blind area.

Exclusion of organic disease

1 Normal pattern visual evoked potentials are very reassuring and an electroretinogram should be performed at the same time to exclude retinal disease in the presence of a normal eye onto which is superadded a non-organic defect. It must be remembered that non-organic defects may be superimposed on organic defects, especially in older children.

2 Neuroimaging may be necessary if the visual evoked potentials are abnormal or if there is a residual degree of uncertainty.

Management

These cases are often difficult to manage. It is important to discuss with the parents that what they are witnessing is a normal stress reaction. It is not a 'naughtiness' of the child, but it is related to some life event either at school or at home and they need to look into this to see if there are any stressing elements.

Often it is very difficult to find a clear-cut stressing disorder and the parents are helped by realising that this is a common reaction and should not be looked on as being significantly abnormal and that the prognosis is generally good.

Although the prognosis is good, there are some children, especially if they have had other stress-related symptoms or if there is a lack of acceptance and insight by the family, or if there is other psychopathology, in whom the symptoms may be prolonged or other systems become involved as vision improves, i.e. the patient may develop a limp or neurological symptom. In these cases a psychiatrist's or psychologist's expert help may be useful.

27: Nystagmus and Eye Movement Disorders

Introduction

Definitions

Nystagmus is a rhythmic oscillation of one or both eyes about one or more axes. The movements may be sinusoidal ('pendular') or with phases of different velocities ('jerk'). Nystagmus can be physiological, i.e. optokinetic, end point and voluntary nystagmus, or pathological. In childhood, pathological nystagmus can be of early onset (before 6 months) or of late onset. Late onset nystagmus is usually of a neurological nature. Early onset nystagmus can be divided into three basic forms, sensory defect, congenital idiopathic or neurological (Fig. 27.1).

Jerk nystagmus = nystagmus with a slow phase and a quick phase of unequal velocity.

Pendular nystagmus = sinusoidal, i.e. with no defined quick or slow phase. Triangular nystagmus may be pendular but, having equal phases of unchanging velocity, it is not sinusoidal. Many forms of nystagmus vary from time to time and from one position of gaze to another, i.e. they may be jerk in one direction and pendular in another.

Axis of oscillation = horizontal, vertical, oblique.

Circumrotary = rotation about multiple axes, i.e. the eye goes round and round if the axes are out of phase or obliquely if the axes are in phase.

Torsional nystagmus = rotation about an anteroposterior axis.

Direction of rotation = direction of fast phase for notational purposes. It is usually the slow phase that reflects the pathology.

Amplitude = length of excursion measured in degrees of the slow or fast phase. 'Fine', 'Medium' 'Coarse'.

Frequency = number of beats per second.

Intensity = amplitude × frequency.

Manifest nystagmus = nystagmus that is present when both eyes are open.

Latent nystagmus = nystagmus that appears when one or both eyes are closed. It is a specific form of nystagmus that may be manifest (see below).

Gaze evoked nystagmus = nystagmus that appears on eccentric gaze but not in primary position.

Asymmetrical and dissociated nystagmus = nystagmus that has different characteristics in the two eyes.

Compound nystagmus = nystagmus which is made up of two or more different types of nystagmus.

Examination and notation of patients with nystagmus

In all cases, a history of the onset, a family history and an examination of any available relatives and a documentation of the progression of the nystagmus and its variations with age, time and lighting conditions, intermittency and the parents' opinion of the child's vision, the presence of photophobia, etc. must be taken.

A full eye examination should include acuity where possible, colour vision, and a slit lamp examination (particularly looking for transillumination in order to detect albinism (Fig. 27.2)). A note should be made of any abnormal head posture and the vision is tested with and without the head posture.

Further investigations

All cases require neurophysiological studies unless they are children who are sufficiently testable and fulfil precisely the criteria for typical congenital idiopathic nystagmus. If the neurophysiological studies are normal, unless the nystagmus is 'neurological' or has a very prominent torsional or circumrotary component, computerized tomography (CT) scanning is not normally required.

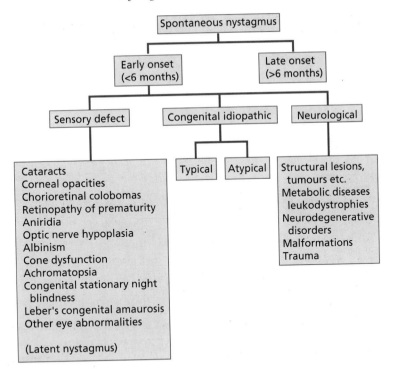

Fig. 27.1 A classification of nystagmus with onset in infancy. The term early onset nystagmus describes all nystagmus with an onset before 6 months and is divided into three: sensory defect nystagnous describes nystagmus associated with demonstrable anterior visual pathway disease including latent nystagmus; congenital idicpatric nystagmus describes nystagmus not associated with any demonstrable visual or neurological impairment (except for poor acuity directly attributable to the nystagmus); neurological nystagmus describes nystagmus not in the other two categories and usually associated with neurological disease.

The flowchart reads:

Spontaneous nystagmus
- **Early onset (<6 months)**
  - **Sensory defect**
    - Cataracts
    - Corneal opacities
    - Chorioretinal colobomas
    - Retinopathy of prematurity
    - Aniridia
    - Optic nerve hypoplasia
    - Albinism
    - Cone dysfunction
    - Achromatopsia
    - Congenital stationary night blindness
    - Leber's congenital amaurosis
    - Other eye abnormalities

    (Latent nystagmus)
  - **Congenital idiopathic**
    - Typical
    - Atypical
- **Late onset (>6 months)**
  - **Neurological**
    - Structural lesions, tumours etc.
    - Metabolic diseases
    - leukodystrophies
    - Neurodegenerative disorders
    - Malformations
    - Trauma

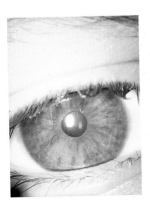
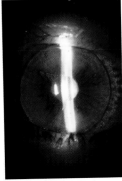

Fig. 27.2 X-linked ocular albinism in a child of Indian origin who presented with nystagmus and poor vision. Showing a brown iris, but marked transillumination.

Documentation

See Figs 27.3 and 27.4.

Physiological forms of nystagmus and their disorders

Optokinetic nystagmus (OKN)

This is a normal response to a moving visual scene with the slow phases in the direction of the scene movement. It is best elicited using a full field but since this is difficult clinically, older children and adults may be asked to view an optokinetic drum or tape. The problem with testing OKN in an infant using a drum or tape is that the child is usually more interested in the tester than he or she is in the target! Nonetheless, a positive response can be helpful. OKN can be suppressed if a stationary object is viewed.

OKN abnormalities occur in.

1 Very poor vision. OKN has been used to quantify visual acuity but it is not a clinically reliable technique.

2 Saccade initiation failure (SIF). SIF (ocular motor apraxia) gives rise to an abnormal OKN in which the eyes deviate towards the side of rotation of the OKN stimulus but there are either absent or abnormal quick phases (see below).

3 Intracranial lesions. OKN abnormalities can occur with acute vestibular or cerebellar disease, occipital disease and occipitoparietal disorders.

4 Congenital idiopathic or sensory-defect nystagmus.

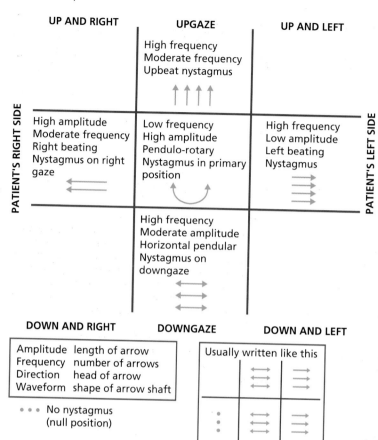

Fig. 27.3 A descriptive way of documenting nystagmus. The notation is mostly for comparison over time. It is difficult with this system to describe torsional nystagmus—it has to be noted separately.

Monocular OKN asymmetry

Infants in the first 6 months of life, but most characteristically neonates, have highly asymmetrical OKN when viewing monocularly. The temporonasal OKN is relatively normal and the nasotemporal OKN is more erratic. This asymmetry declines over about 6 months, even longer at high stimulus speeds. With early disruption of vision, especially binocular vision, the OKN asymmetry persists and may become permanent (Fig. 27.5).

The vestibulo-ocular reflex (VOR) and vestibular nystagmus

Eye movements occur in response to rotation of the head in the light or dark, they are generated by the semicircular canals and their function is to maintain the position of the eyes despite movements of the head and body. Acute or severe loss leads to oscillopsia on any movement, and poor vision due to the inability to stabilize retinal images during body and head movements. Even sitting in a car may be very unpleasant.

The VOR can be induced by rapidly turning the child's head up or down (doll's head manoeuvre) or by rotation in a chair or, with an infant, by holding the child at arms' length while rotating around in a chair or while standing. In the light the responses are of combination of optokinetic response and vestibular ocular responses and in the dark it is purely vestibular. When rotation stops there may be 1 or 2 beats of after-nystagmus. In the laboratory, the VOR is tested in the dark using a rotating chair.

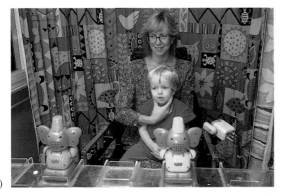

(a)

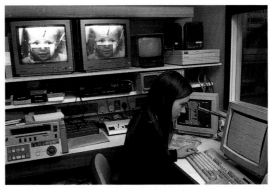

(b)

Fig. 27.4 The eye movement laboratory at Great Ormond Street Hospital.

(a) Horizontal eye movements are measured by electrodes placed at the outer canthus of each eye and a ground electrode at the mid-forehead position; a monocular recording can be made with an electrode on the inner canthus, and vertical eye movements can be measured by placing electrodes above and below an eye. The infant sits on a carer's lap with the head held still and any nystagmus is examined in the cardinal gaze positions. Each eye is patched in turn and the viewing eye is abducted and adducted to reveal any latent nystagmus or latent component. Full-field binocular and monocular optokinetic testing is achieved with a brightly coloured attractive curtain that completely encircles the patient and is rotated at various speeds. Saccades are readily elicited by large noisy toys from the very young, or by small lights or LEDs from the older child. Vestibular nystagmus is induced by completely darkening the room and rotating the chair at a constant speed in each direction. The patient is monitored at all times by an infrared camera.

(b) The video image and electro-oculographic signals are relayed to the adjacent room for recording and superimposed, allowing the eye movement trace and the visual appearance of the eyes to be examined simultaneously.

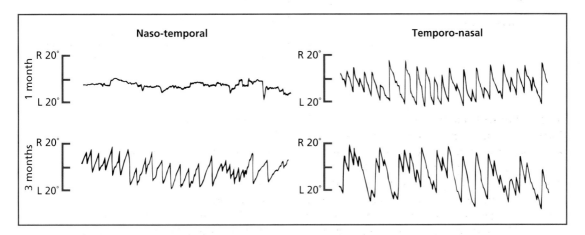

Fig. 27.5 OKN elicited by a full-field curtain from a healthy infant viewing monocularly with the right eye. At 1 month of age a normal OKN can be elicited with slow phases in the temporo-nasal direction of the viewing eye (i.e. to the left), but there is no response in the naso-temporal direction. Normally by 3 months, the naso-temporal OKN has much improved, but will persist with early-onset uniocular visual deficits.

Abnormalities of the VOR occur in the following situations.

1 Cerebellar abnormalities give rise to a high gain, i.e. large amplitude eye movements in response to movement. Absent quick phases occur in SIF (see below) and the VOR is abnormal in children, infants in particular, with sensory defect nystagmus or congenital idiopathic nystagmus. Prolonged optokinetic after-nystagmus occurs in children who are blind or those who have cerebellar disease.

2 When the head moves there is an automatic equal and opposite eye movement. Therefore, to move the head and the eyes together, the VOR must be suppressed. It is thought to have the same mechanism as smooth pursuit and abnormalities of it occur in a variety of diseases, in particular cerebellar disorders. It is elicited by getting the child to fixate an object that is rotating with the head, i.e. a pin stuck in a wooden tongue depressor which is held in the teeth. Normally, the child can follow the pin without eliciting nystagmus but, if the VOR suppression is abnormal, nystagmus occurs.

3 Acute lesions of the vestibular apparatus and its central connections gives rise to a compound nystagmus that has a prominent torsional component. In peripheral disease, the horizontal slow phases are towards the side of the lesion.

Circularvection, a sensation of self-rotation, dizziness, and oscillopsia are common, but usually transient. Bilateral lesions are more severe and take a longer time to recover.

End point nystagmus

Many people have a small amplitude jerk nystagmus when they look far to one side and are not associated to any other neurological signs or eye movement abnormalities.

Voluntary nystagmus

Since about 5% of the population can imitate nystagmus voluntarily this could be considered as being normal. Usually it is a high frequency, low amplitude nystagmus that is mostly horizontal (vertical and circumrotary nystagmus are much more difficult to perform and voluntary torsional nystagmus is unknown). It is usually associated with convergence and pupil constriction and often by facial tics and grimacing. Normally it cannot be sustained for more than a few seconds. It is effectively pendular with both phases being quick, i.e. 'back to back' saccades.

Latent and manifest latent nystagmus

Latent nystagmus is usually observed within the first few years of life, occasionally in the first few months. It is common and it occurs in association with early onset visual disorders and strabismus. Latent nystagmus is visible only when one or both eyes are covered. It may become manifest, i.e. manifest latent nystagmus, when there is poor vision in one eye such as when an amblyopic eye is trying to fix or when there is an organic visual defect such as a cataract or corneal opacity. Both latent nystagmus and manifest latent nystagmus are jerk forms of nystagmus with the fast phases in the direction of the uncovered or fixing eye. It becomes more intense when the fixing eye abducts and less intense when it adducts. This sometimes results in an abnormal head posture. It has characteristic decelerating or linear slow phases (Fig. 27.6).

Latent nystagmus is very often associated with dissociated vertical deviation.

In itself, latent or manifest latent nystagmus does not usually require treatment but if there is a marked abnormal head posture associated with it, usually due to the fixing eye being held in adduction, a recession of the medial rectus of the fixing eye associated with appropriate surgery to maintain alignment of the non-fixing eye, may help. Injection of *Botulinus* toxin into the medial rectus may help to predict the value of surgery in these cases.

Congenital idiopathic nystagmus (CIN) and early onset sensory defect nystagmus (SDN)

These are forms of nystagmus that may not be distinguishable from each other and that have an early onset. SDN is secondary to a diagnosable sensory defect whilst in CIN it is not possible clinically to make such a diagnosis. Many cases that were thought to be CIN have been found to be SDN when appropriate investigations were carried out. CIN is sometimes called 'motor' nystagmus but,

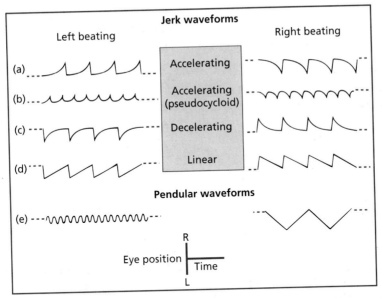

Fig. 27.6 Stylized waveform types seen in horizontal nystagmus for left beating (left column) and right beating (right column). By convention up = right, and down = left. (a) Accelerating slow phases (increasing velocity slow phases), where the speed of the eye increase with time during the slow phase; seen in CIN/SDN. (b) A common variant of the ASP waveform, called 'pseudocycloid'. (c) Decelerating slow phases (decreasing velocity slow phases) seen in latent nystagmus. (d) Linear or constant velocity slow phases where speed does not change during the slow phase. (e) Pendular nystagmus (i.e. no quick phases), with sinusoidal waveform (left) and triangular waveform (right).

usually, no ocular or other movement defect can be found.

CIN and SDN cannot be distinguished by analysis of any of the features of the nystagmus itself and in the child of less than 3 or 4 years, further investigation is almost invariably required.

Clinically, 'typical' CIN is characterized by a purely horizontal nystagmus in all positions of gaze with clinically normal eyes in a child who in all aspects is developing normally. It does not require further investigation in a verbal child who can be adequately tested or when there is a family history of CIN.

Any waveform other than purely horizontal and any other failure to meet the criteria of typical congenital idiopathic nystagmus (i.e. optic atrophy, photophobia, developmental delay, etc.) should force the clinician to investigate the child with neurophysiology and possibly CT scanning; this 'atypical' CIN, neurological nystagmus and SDN often cannot be told apart clinically from examination of the eye movements which are much more diverse in their manifestations, they may have vertical, oblique, torsional or compound waveforms.

SDN is usually suspected on clinical grounds by history and examination.

- Poor vision.
- Ophthalmoscopically visible retinal or optic nerve defects.
- Photophobia (cone dystrophy).
- Abnormal pupil reactions (retinal and optic nerve disease).
- High refractive error (retinal disease).
- Family history of a visual defect or consanguinity.
- Developmental delay, seizures or other central nervous system signs.

Analysis of the waveform does not help to distinguish CIN from SDN, but the presence of horizontal accelerating slow phases is characteristic of early onset SDN/CIN, thus distinguishing it from neurological nystagmus. Accelerating slow phases, however, are not always present (Fig. 27.7).

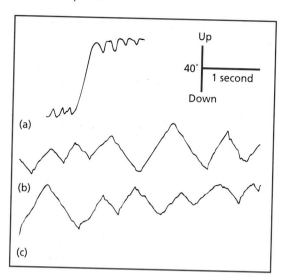

Fig. 27.7 Actual waveforms recorded by electro-oculography. (a) Typical accelerating slow phase nystagmus recorded from a 3 year old with CIN, showing leftward beats in left gaze and rightward beats in right gaze. (b) Large amplitude low frequency triangular pendular nystagmus recorded from an albino infant aged 3 months. (c) Same infant as (b) but recorded during full-field optokinetic stimulation. Nystagmus remains essentially unaltered (calibration approximate).

The amplitude of CIN/SDN often varies with age, even being undetectable in the first month or two, increasing rapidly in the next few months only to decrease after 6–12 months. The amplitude may vary with fatigue, illness, drug treatment or stress.

Vision in CIN is usually relatively good. It is usual for the child to have better than 6/36 acuity. It is most frequently in the order of 6/24–6/9. Oscillopsia does not occur unless abnormal visual circumstances are induced such as holding the eye steady or occasionally transiently after surgery. Colour vision is normal. They should have undoubtedly normal optic discs. Astigmatism or other refractive errors are acceptable as being a part of CIN and the child should be developmentally completely normal.

CIN may be inherited as an autosomal dominant trait but usually there is no family history. Other forms of inheritance are unusual.

The vision in SDN depends on the causative condition

Adaptive strategies in CIN/SDN

Abnormal head posture

In many cases of CIN, and sometimes in SDN, the child adopts an abnormal head posture, especially when trying hard to view an object. The head is held in such a position that the eyes are in the null zone, i.e. where the nystagmus intensity is least. The head turn is usually horizontal but occasionally a chin up or chin down position is maintained or even a tilt.

Surgery to reduce the head posture can be carried out. For instance, if the null position is to the left and therefore the head posture to the right, the aim is to shift the eyes relatively to the right, i.e. recess the right medial rectus and the left lateral rectus and resect the right lateral rectus and the left medial rectus. The main problem is that, to achieve long term success, large amounts of surgery may have to be carried out, usually resulting in gaze limitation and the operations should be restricted to persons who have substantial problems as a result of the abnormal head posture. An explanation to the parents and to the child's schoolteachers that the head posture is an adaptive strategy from which the child gains and a description of the high recurrence rate following surgery should be mandatory.

Visual acuity is not significantly improved by the surgery.

Box 27.1 Surgical treatment of abnormal head postures in patients with nystagmus

Examples
1 Large R+R to fixing eye only in manifest latent nystagmus (MLN) with esotropia
   Blind left eye, left esotropia 30 D, manifest latent nystagmus with null zone to left, AHP to right: R MR recession 6–7 mm, R LR resection 8 mm.
2 Bilateral asymmetrical R+R in CIN with exotropia.
   L exotropia 25 D, L VA 20/100, R VA 20/20 AHP 30 degrees to R, nullzone to left:
   R LR resection 9 mm, R MR recession 7 mm;
   L MR resection 11 mm, L LR recession 12 mm.
3 Bilateral R+R in CIN with no strabismus.
   CIN, no strabismus, VA 20/40 R+L, 100 seconds of arc stereoacuity, null zone to left, AHP 40 degrees to R:
   R LR resection 10 mm, R MR recession 8 mm;
   L MR resection 9 mm, L LR recession 10 mm.

Other treatments for abnormal head postures

Either Fresnel, glass or plastic prisms can also be used to shift the eyes in relation to the head. They are only practicable for small head turns because glass or plastic prisms are too thick and Fresnel prisms are subject to distortion and chromatic aberration when higher powers are used.

Surgery to reduce the nystagmus amplitude

Surgery can be carried out directed at the nystagmus itself by very large recession of all four horizontal muscles. This technique has not yet been fully evaluated and is unlikely to have long-term benefits.

Head shaking in CIN

Head shaking may occur with any form of nystagmus but most typically with CIN: it occurs in two main situations.

1 As an adaptive strategy to achieve better acuity because:

(a) the shaking itself, whether it is vertical or horizontal, in some way suppresses the nystagmus; probably the VOR induced by the shaking suppresses the nystagmus and 'overrides' it; and

(b) the VOR may be manipulated so that the movement of the head, instead of inducing an exactly equal and opposite eye movement, in some way counters the movement of the eye so that the eye in space stays relatively still or at least there are plateaus of steadiness within the nystagmus waveform, thus improving the acuity.

These forms of head shake occur when the child is trying to look hard at an object, and when seen in an infant, imply a relatively good prognosis.

2 Head shaking may occur as a head tremor of common genesis to the nystagmus, i.e. the head shake and the nystagmus have the same cause.

Other forms of treatment for CIN

Drugs, auditory biofeedback (the patient hears auditory signals related to the amplitude of the nystagmus so that the patient knows when his or her nystagmus intensity is least) and contact lenses, as a form of feedback from touch via the eyelids have all been tried. Treatment with drugs is not usually recommended although baclofen has been used with some effect in patients with periodic alternating nystagmus.

> **Box 27.2 Head oscillations in children**
>
> **1** Shaking or nodding.
> (a) With congenital idiopathic nystagmus:
> VOR suppressing the nystagmus;
> summation of head and eye movements giving plateaus of eye steadiness;
> nystagmus and head shaking of common genesis.
> (b) Spasmus nutans (see below).
> (c) Bobble-headed doll syndrome. This is a to-and-fro bobbing of the head reminiscent of that of a doll's. Since it is often seen with hydrocephalus and third ventricular tumours, there is not infrequently a sensory defect or neurological nystagmus.
> (d) With sensory defect or neurological nystagmus.
> (e) Ocular bobbing, reverse ocular bobbing and ocular dipping. These are eye movements seen mostly with widespread brain disease and sometimes localized pontine disease with vertical eye movements with a fast and a slow phase. Most of the patients are comatose and these are poor prognostic signs.
> **2** Head thrusts associated with saccade initiation failure (SIF, congenital oculomotor apraxia). These are seen as compensation for abnormal saccade movements (see Saccade initiation failure).

Spasmus nutans

The nature of this eye and head movement disorder is between a form of neurological nystagmus (see below) and atypical CIN; it is a retrospective diagnosis and can occasionally be mimicked by a number of pathological conditions in particular nystagmus associated with chiasmal glioma. It is a self-limiting condition with an onset from a few months up to 2 years with the following features.

1 Asymmetrical pendular nystagmus. The nystagmus in one eye may be of greater amplitude and even a different direction to the other eye. This is usually the first sign noticed by the parents.

2 Head nodding. This may be vertical, horizontal or compound and is often intermittent.

3 An abnormal head posture.

The diagnosis of spasmus nutans demands investigation with neurophysiology and sometimes by CT scanning.

Neurological nystagmus

Any acquired nystagmus in childhood requires investigation because it often has associations with underlying neurological disease. There are many forms of nystagmus which can be identified clinically but eye movement studies and recordings play a significant role in identifying them.

Gaze-paretic nystagmus

Gaze-paretic nystagmus occurs on eccentric gaze to fast phases in the direction of gaze. It may be horizontal, vertical or oblique or any combination of these.
- It is due to a mismatch between gaze-holding circuitry of the brainstem and cerebellum and the dynamics of the extraocular muscles.
- Often associated with other cerebellar or brainstem signs.
- Often bilateral.
- When unilateral beats towards the side of the lesion.
- May be drug-induced.
- Occurs in vestibulo-cerebellar disorders.
- Frequent in muscle disease including myasthenia.

Rebound nystagmus

Rebound nystagmus is gaze-paretic nystagmus which reduces in amplitude or reverses beat on sustained eccentric gaze. It is associated with a variety of cerebellar diseases

Acquired pendular nystagmus (APN)
- High frequency.
- Low amplitude.
- Vertical, horizontal or compound which may be asymmetrical.
- Pendular in all gaze directions.
- Optokinetic responses present (in contrast to SDN/CIN).
- APN is non-localizing.

APN occurs with the following:
- Demyelinating disease.
- Oculopalatal myoclonus (synchronous oscillations of the palate, head and eyes).
- Drug intoxication.
- Neurodegenerative diseases.
- APN may be significantly asymmetrical, similar to spasmus nutans (see above).

See-saw nystagmus
- Usually moderate amplitude, moderate frequency, one eye elevates and intorts as the other depresses and extorts.
- Often asymmetrical, the eye with the worse vision having the largest amplitude.
- Classically associated with chiasmal and hypothalamic diseases and a bitemporal hemianiopia.
- Glioma, craniopharyngioma commonest causes.
- Rarely idiopathic or associated with achiasmia, optic nerve hypoplasia, midbrain or retinal disease.

Vestibular nystagmus
See above.

Positional nystagmus
- Nystagmus elicited by head movement.
- Peripheral vestibular disorders.
- Espisodic vertigo.
- In childhood, usually secondary to labyrinthitis or trauma.

Downbeat nystagmus
- Fast phases downwards.
- Amplitude usually increases on downgaze, especially down and lateral gaze.
- May intensify with convergence.
- Associated with other eye movement defects.
- Causes:
  (a) craniocervical junction abnormalities, i.e. Arnold–Chiari malformation basilar invagination, syringobulbia, glioma, etc;
  (b) cerebellar degenerations;
  (c) raised intracranial pressure;
  (d) drugs, anticonvulsants, lithium and alcohol;
  (e) occasionally seen as a transient phenomenon in a normal infant.

Upbeat nystagmus
- Fast phases upwards, increases on upgaze.
- May become oblique on up and lateral gaze.
- Causes:
    (a) cerebellar degeneration;
    (b) drugs;
    (c) familial, autosomal dominant (a form of CIN);
    (d) organophosphate poisoning;
    (e) pontomedullary abnormalities.

Periodic alternating nystagmus (PAN)

This is a cyclic phenomenon in which there is a horizontal jerk nystagmus that spontaneously reverses direction, the periodicity of which ranges from 60 to 180 seconds.

Causes:
    (a) congenital or acquired;
    (b) if acquired usually associated with cerebellar or brainstem diseases;
    (c) drug intoxication;
    (d) visual loss;
    (e) associated with congenital idiopathic nystagmus;
    (f) frequent in albinos when studied by electronystagmography.

Baclofen treatment may help

Other cyclic eye movement phenomena

Periodic alternating gaze deviation

This is a phenomenon related to PAN in which there is a conjugate eye deviation periodically alternating between one side and the other, usually associated with a saccade palsy.

Ping-pong gaze

A constant reversal of direction of the eyes, usually every few seconds, usually associated with severe neurological development disorders.

Convergence-retraction nystagmus
See below.

Saccade abnormalities

Saccades are rapid eye movements used to shift gaze. Fast phases of nystagmus are saccadic.

Saccades are generated by ipsilateral burst cells in the pons in response to supranuclear excitation. Simultaneously, pause cells are inhibited (Fig. 27.8).

Saccade initiation failure (SIF)—'congenital oculomotor apraxia'

This is most frequently seen as a congenital defect of voluntary saccades.

Patients present in different ways depending on the severity and their age.
- As an apparently blind infant: the lack of rapid movements and the inability to shift gaze to an object of interest leads parents to think that their child cannot see, especially before the baby has head control and can initiate head thrusts.
- Because of the head thrusts or blinking (see below).
- Because of difficulties at school.

Most frequently, only horizontal saccades are involved, occasionally vertical saccades. SIF is intermittently brought out when the child is trying to look very hard to one or the other side. It is usually idiopathic but has been described in association with congenital brain malformations, most frequently agenesis of the corpus callosum and cerebellar vermis hypoplasia.

It may occur in association with a variety of neurodegenerative conditions, in particular infantile Gaucher's disease, Niemann–Pick type C, ataxia telangiectasia, various spinocerebellar degenerations, perinatal problems, posterior fossa tumours and other acquired disorders. In these cases vertical saccades are usually affected.

To make up for the inability to initiate saccades, children adopt a variety of strategies:

1 Head thrusts. The head is thrust towards the side that the child is trying to look at, the eyes move by the VOR in the opposite direction until they reach extreme gaze when they are dragged towards the direction the child wants to look, sometimes two or three thrusts may be needed. Once the eye has achieved its target the head may return to the mid-position.

2 Blink-saccade synkinesis. Saccades seem to be facilitated by blinking. The child makes a blink at

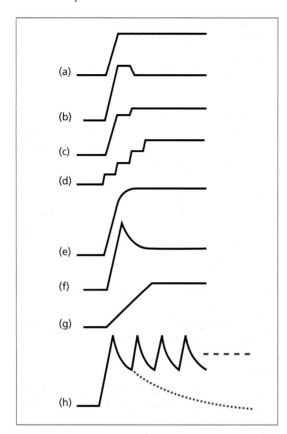

Fig. 27.8 Saccadic dysmetria.
(a) Normometria—the target is reached in a single accurate saccade.
(b) Cerebellar disease with 'gain hypermetria'—the saccade overshoots the target and requires a secondary saccade in the opposite direction.
(c) Hypometria—the saccade undershoots the target, requiring a secondary corrective saccade in the same direction.
(d) Severe hypometria with multiple corrective saccades. This is normal in the first few months of life.
(e) Pulse-step mismatch 1. Pulse hypometria; when the pulse command is too small to reach the target, the end of the saccade is slow because it is driven only by the step signal.
(f) Pulse-step mismatch 2. Pulse hypermetria; when the pulse is too large for the target the eyes overshoot the target and drift back to it without an intersaccadic interval.
(g) Slow saccades (see text).
(h) Neural integrator failure. Since the tonic signal to maintain the step (to hold the eye in the eccentric position) is defective the eyes drift back to the primary position (dotted line). In an attentive patient with a partial lesion there is an attempt to re-foveate the target which gives rise to gaze-paretic nystagmus.

the time that the saccade is initiated, sometimes moving the head at the same time.
3 Other strategies. If vertical movements are normal, the child may tilt his head to shift horizontal gaze with vertical movements, sometimes reading is achieved by moving the book rather than the eyes.

Investigation and management
Most cases can be detected clinically. The head thrusts or the blink-saccade synkinesis may be seen or the child may simply not make rapid horizontal movements. One of the easiest ways to elicit the abnormality is to pick up the small baby and spin him round, or spin the older child round in a chair. This will bring about a combination of OKN and VOR and the eyes, lacking a fast-phase to the nystagmus 'lock up' in lateral gaze, opposite to the direction of rotation.

Although most children with SIF are healthy and do not have any development problems, a substantial proportion are clumsy, and some may have educational difficulties beyond any purely motor problems. Liaison with the school may be very helpful to the child.

Slow saccades
Saccades with abnormally low velocity are usually due to defects in the brainstem saccade generator neurones. They occur in the conditions listed below.
- Olivopontocerebellar atrophy.
- Spinocerebellar degenerations.
- Progressive supranuclear palsy.
- Brainstem palsies.
- Neurodegenerative diseases.
- Drug toxicity.
- Internuclear ophthamoplegia (see below).
- Ocular muscle disease:
    (a) myasthenia gravis;
    (b) mitochondrial cytopathy.
- Slow saccades occur in normal sleepy patients.

Fast saccades
- Rare.
- May occur with acute cerebellar disease, i.e. opsoclonus.
- Transient in myasthenia.

Intrusive saccades
Square-wave jerks
These are small amplitude, short latency eye movements that occur in both light and dark. Their amplitude is up to 10 degrees. They are involuntary deviations from the point of fixation followed by an interval (the 'intersaccadic interval') of about 150–200 ms, followed by a corrective saccade back to the target. Small amplitude square wave jerks occur in normals, larger ones occur in cerebellar disorders and a variety of other neurological diseases.

Ocular flutter
These are bursts of horizontal eye movements with no intersaccadic interval (this suggests that they are 'preprogrammed' and not altered by visual input). They may occur immediately after a saccade (flutter dysmetria).

They are most frequently seen in association with acute cerebellar encephalitis and related to exanthemas, particularly varicella.

Opsoclonus
Opsoclonus is characterized by bursts of large amplitude, multidirectional eye movements. There can be many oscillations in each burst and the trajectories are often multiplanar or chaotic. The child may have other cerebellar abnormalities, ataxia, etc., in which case it is sometimes called 'Opsoclonus–Polymyoclonus'.

Aetiology
Idiopathic. This is often known as 'Dancing Eyes and Dancing Feet' syndrome. It is usually self-limited and may be improved by adrenocorticotropic hormone or steroids. There is often a residual neurological deficit.

Neuroblastoma-associated. Opsoclonus occurs in association with neuroblastoma which is usually occult. The presence of opsoclonus carries a favourable prognosis for the neuroblastoma.

Encephalitis/meningitis. A variety of causes of acute meningitis or encephalitis may be associated with opsoclonus.

- Undetermined aetiology.
- Post-exanthemas.
- Polioencephalitis.
- Coxsackie B3, St Louis encephalitis.
- Others.

Other acute cerebellar disease or intoxications—Neonatal. Opsoclonus has been described in otherwise normal neonates. It may also be associated with neonatal problems.

Macrosaccadic oscillations
These are deviations of the eyes with a 150–200 ms intersaccadic interval which increase and then decrease in amplitude; they are seen in acute cerebellar disease.

Saccadic accuracy disorders (dysmetria)
Hypometria (see Fig. 27.8)
In this, the saccade falls short of the target and secondary saccades are necessary.

Hypermetria
The saccade overshoots the target and secondary saccades in the opposite direction are needed to achieve the target.

Hypometria is normal in large amplitude saccades, especially in young children, but dysmetric saccades occur in cerebellar disease, brainstem disease, visual field defects (hypometria into the blind field), muscle disease (mostly hypometria but in myasthenia some saccades may be hypermetric), in oculomotor apraxia and in basal ganglia disease.

Neural integrator failure (Fig. 27.9)
During the generation of a saccade, a velocity command to the burst cells gives rise to a pulse of increased excitation which results in the rapid part of the eye movement. To hold the eye in the new position, the velocity command needs to be integrated via a 'neural integrator' into the step position command. If the neural integrator is defective, the step position command is abnormal and the eye drifts back towards the primary position. If the neural integrator time constant is low, the eye drifts back more quickly so eccentric gaze holding is

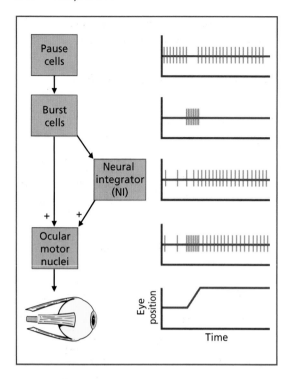

Fig. 27.9 The role of the neural integrator in generating saccades. Tonic pause neurones are inhibited by a high-level triggering signal: this disinhibits burst units, which then fire rapidly to give an intense *phasic* signal that is transmitted via the appropriate oculomotor nuclei to the agonist extraocular muscle, while the antagonist muscle is inhibited. Simultaneously the burst signal is passed to the neural integrator which 'counts' the spikes in the burst, integrates them, and generates a new signal that is appropriate for the new eye *position*. This tonic signal is also to the extra-ocular muscles via the oculomotor nuclei and it holds the eye steady at the end of a saccade.

more difficult. Usually, the neural integrator defect is partial: this results in gaze-paretic nystagmus, more severe disease may result in an inability to hold any lateral gaze. It is associated particularly with cerebellar flocculus and paraflocculus disorders.

Antisaccades

Antisaccades are saccades produced in a test situation that are made in the opposite direction to a rapidly presented stimulus. It is a test of high-level control saccadic eye movements and may be abnor-mal in basal ganglia disease or widespread cerebral disorders.

Smooth pursuit

Smooth pursuit occurs when the eyes smoothly follow a smoothly moving visual target. Smooth pursuit may share the same neural substrate as VOR suppression.

Smooth pursuit is tested by attracting the child's attention to a slowly moving interesting target, horizontally and vertically, with the head held still. Abnormalities occur in visual defects, cortical and cerebellar lesions, drug intoxication and in delayed visual maturation.

Vergence

Vergence is the ability to change the angle between the visual axes. In convergence the visual axes are brought to bear from a distant to a near object and in divergence the visual axes are brought to bear from a near to a distant object.

Vergence abnormalities are very important in the genesis and management of strabismus.

Divergence paralysis

Divergence paralysis is a convergent strabismus for distance more than near. Sometimes it is associated with an abduction weakness and may be an early manifestation of unilateral or bilateral sixth nerve palsy.

Convergence insufficiency

This is a difficulty in achieving near fixation; there is often an exophoria for near fixation on the cover test. When the child is instructed to converge, the convergence associated pupillary movements are not seen, rather as a lack of drive rather than end-organ failure.

Any underlying psychological problems need to be analysed and, where possible, modified. The symptoms are treated by near-point exercises in which the child is instructed to hold at arms' length an object with some detail on it (such as a wooden tongue depressor onto which has been stuck small letters or figures). The target so formed is gradually moved closer to the child's eye and he is instructed to keep it single and clear: as soon as it becomes blurred or double the target is moved away a little and the cycle is repeated. The child needs strong encouragement to concentrate on the treatment to get the best effect. Only very rarely is surgery in the form of medial rectus resection indicated.

Convergence paralysis, with a tropia in primary position may be due to midbrain disease.

Spasm of the near reflex

This is a non-organic problem which usually occurs in older children or young adults, in which episodic blurred and double vision occur with the patient complaining of eye ache and asthenopia. The convergence is associated with pupillary constriction. It may last for several minutes. It is rarely caused by organic disease but midbrain lesions, toxicity and cyclic oculomotor palsy have been described as underlying causes. Treatment is difficult. A psychological evaluation is important but often fails to show any clear-cut problem, or any problem that can be treated. Sometimes the symptoms can be improved by cycloplegia with atropine, the reading difficulty so caused is treated with bifocal spectacles. Sometimes, miotics such as pilocarpine may help. The symptoms are often prolonged for several months.

Vergence abnormalities in midbrain lesions (the Sylvian aqueduct or Parinaud's syndromes)

In dorsal midbrain disease there may be convergence paralysis and rarely convergence spasm. It is usually associated with:

- convergence retraction nystagmus: these are high velocity adducting movements usually on attempted upgaze. They are faster than true convergence movements and may be associated with discomfort;
- light-near dissociation of the pupil reactions;
- limitation of upgaze;
- lid retraction (Collier's sign);
- skew deviation:
  - (a) a vertical supranuclear disorder
  - (b) comitant or non-comitant
  - (c) intorsion of the elevated eye

- (d) extorsion of the depressed eye; and
- vertical, especially downbeat, nystagmus.

Localizing ocular motor signs

Medulla

- Downbeat nystagmus.
- Periodic alternating nystagmus.
- Torsional nystagmus.
- Gaze paretic and rebound nystagmus.
- Wallenberg's lateral medullary syndrome (posterior inferior cerebellar artery occlusion usually in the elderly):
  - (a) vertigo;
  - (b) facial and corneal anaesthesia;

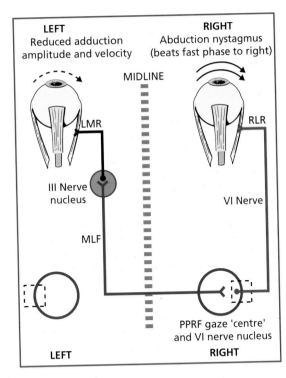

Fig. 27.10 Pontine disease: INO and gaze abnormalities. To achieve gaze to the right, supranuclear signals to the right pontine paramedian reticular formation (PPRF) cause excitation of the right VI nerve nucleus which causes the right eye to move to the right. Signals from the PPRF go to the left medial rectus muscle, via the MLF, and the left eye moves to the right. An INO involves the MLF, and the 'one and a half' syndrome involves the MLF and the PPRF (see text).

(c) lateropulsion, a sensation of being pulled to the side of the lesion;

(d) saccadic hypermetria, ipsilateral to the lesion (overshooting of the eyes towards the side of the lesion);

(e) saccadic hypometria, contralateral to the lesion.

Pons

- Gaze palsies:

    (a) ipsilateral gaze-evoked nystagmus, reduced amplitude and velocity of ipsilateral saccades; these may be congenital (syndromes of brainstem dysplasia including Mobius and related disorders) or acquired (see INO causes below).

- Internuclear ophthalmoplegia (INO) (Fig. 27.10):

    (a) unilateral or bilateral;

    (b) lesion of the medial longitudinal fasciculus (MLF);

    (c) reduced amplitude and velocity of adduction movements (particularly saccades) towards the side of the lesion. Vergence movements may be preserved in caudal lesions not involving the third nerve nucleus;

    (d) nystagmus of the abducting eye opposite to the lesion;

    (e) skew deviation;

    (f) vertical gaze defects and nystagmus;

    (g) causes:

        (i) demyelating disease:
        multiple sclerosis;
        irradiation;
        (ii) developmental anomalies:
        Arnold–Chiari malformation;
        A-V malformations;
        (iii) tumours;
        (iv) vascular disease;
        (v) encephalitis:
        post-exanthematous;
        viral or bacterial;
        (vi) metabolic disease:
        Maple syrup urine disease;
        a-betalipoproteinuria;
        Fabry's disease.

- 'One-and-a-half' syndrome:

    (a) ipsilateral horizontal gaze palsy and INO due to a combined lesion of the gaze centre and MLF;

    (b) often exotropic, 'paralytic pontine exotropia';

    (c) ipsilateral horizontal gaze palsy, preserved contralateral abduction;

    (d) horizontal ipsilateral slow saccades in partial or resolving lesions;

    (e) causes similar to INO.

- Sixth nerve palsies.

Midbrain

- 'Setting sun' sign:

    (a) acute hydrocephalus;

    (b) due to intrinsic posterior commissure lesions;

    (c) upward saccade failure;

    (d) upgaze palsy with intact lid retraction.

- Dorsal midbrain syndrome (see above).

- Vertical gaze defects and gaze evoked nystagmus.

Cerebellum

- Widespread abnormal eye movements.
- Saccadic smooth pursuit.
- Saccadic dysmetria.
- Gaze paretic and rebound nystagmus.
- Downbeat nystagmus and PAN.

Basal ganglia

- Hypometria of voluntary saccades.
- 'Lock up' of the VOR and OKN.
- Slow saccades.
- Abnormal antisaccades.
- Associated with involuntary movements, dystonia and psychiatric disturbances.

Cerebral cortex

- Searching hypometric saccades into hemianopic field.
- Saccadic pursuit and poor OKN for stimulus movement in the direction ipsilateral to the lesion.
- Transient gaze deviation towards the side of an acute destructive lesion, away from the side in a chronic lesion.
- Transient tonic gaze deviation away from the side of an 'irritative' lesion, with seizures affecting the side of the body toward which the eyes deviate.

Index